# HEADWAY LIFEGUIDES

# TAI CHI

## Robert Parry

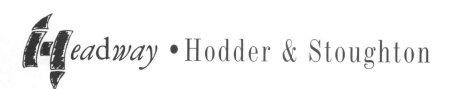
eadway • Hodder & Stoughton

Tai chi is an excellent preventative therapy and a good way of assisting recovery. In times of illness, however, always seek professional medical advice.

The author and publishers would like to thank Christina Jansen for the cover photograph, Roddy Paine for the commissioned photographs, Philip Bannister for the composite diagram on pages 112–115, Annabel Milne for the drawing on page 5, and Taurus Graphics for the drawings on pages 105, 109 and 110.

*Cataloguing in Publication Data is available from the British Library*

ISBN 0 340 60008 X

First published 1994
Impression number   10   9   8   7   6   5   4   3   2   1
Year                          1998   1997   1996   1995   1994

Typeset by Wearset, Boldon, Tyne and Wear.
Printed in Great Britain for Hodder & Stoughton Educational, a division of Hodder Headline Plc, Mill Road, Dunton Green, Sevenoaks, Kent TN13 2YA by Thomson Litho Ltd, East Kilbride.

# CONTENTS

*To my teachers and all those who have shared their knowledge along the way. And to Ruby.*

# INTRODUCTION

Tai chi is many things to different people. The beautiful, controlled and yet freely flowing movements have for centuries inspired men and women from all walks of life, people of all ages and all levels of fitness. Vitality, relaxation, tranquillity, enhanced personal creativity and a sense of purpose – these are just some of tai chi's enduring gifts to the world.

As a shiatsu therapist, I often see people who believe they are relaxed and yet they have in fact never known what it feels like to be relaxed in their body, let alone their mind. This interference through tension and stress with the body's natural healing process is perhaps one of the greatest misfortunes of our times and it is in a bid to help combat this situation – in no matter how small a way – that this book has been written.

In these pages we will be looking exclusively at the health and relaxation aspects of this ancient and yet thoroughly modern art, with step-by-step instructions on how to learn and perform a basic sequence of Yang style tai chi. Don't worry if you have only limited leisure time. Your study can easily be integrated into a normal lifestyle. All it takes is ten minutes each day to get results. And it really is worth it. In the east, exercise systems like tai chi are very popular; they are undertaken in a spirit of moderation and realism and this book urges you to do likewise. Simply do what you can, with the time available – then go ahead and enjoy it!

Although it is not possible to learn tai chi entirely from a book, it is certainly a good way to start and a book can provide that all-important quality of inspiration at any time. Allowing the magic of tai chi to enter your life means being open to the currents and forces of nature, within yourself and within the world around you. It is a journey of a kind, which has to start somewhere. Why not here?

> 66 *A tree the size of a fathom*
> *grows from a blade as thin as a hair.*
> *A tower nine stories high*
> *is built from a small heap of earth.*
> *A journey of a thousand miles*
> *starts in front of your feet . . .* 99
>
> From the ancient Taoist classic *The Tao Te Ching*
> (Sixth century BC)

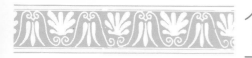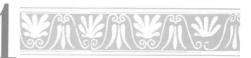

# 1

# BACKGROUND

## What does 'tai chi' mean?

The term 'tai chi' refers not merely to a system of physical exercise. It comes from the ancient Chinese philosophy of Taoism. 'Tao' means 'the way', 'the path' – a universal concept, implying conscious thought and participation. 'Chi' is 'life-force' or 'vital energy' and 'tai' means 'great'. Tai chi, then, is a way of finding yourself and your own special path through life. In classical Chinese literature such as the *I Ching*, sections of which date back as far as the twelfth century BC, we are told of a state of harmony that exists in all of nature – and this is called *The Tai Chi*. It is also often pictured as a symbol called *The Tai Chi T'u* (Fig. 1).

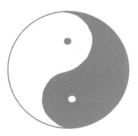

*Fig. 1    The Tai Chi T'u symbol*

This is sometimes also called the 'double-fish diagram', because it looks a little like two fishes chasing each other's tails. Clearly what we have here is a circle, divided equally into a light and a dark sector. These are called the 'Yang' and the 'Yin' respectively. You will have noticed that the division between Yang and Yin is not just a straight line; it is a graceful curve, suggesting movement and the interplay of opposites. Light (or Yang) changes into darkness (Yin) and then back to light again. Note, also, the eye, or seed, of each opposite located deep within each sector, indicating still further the possibilities of change and transformation.

You can probably think of other examples of Yang and Yin in the world around you: day and night; summer and winter; hot and cold; the positive and negative force of electricity; advancing and retreating armies, or the rise and fall of empires both personal and global. All this is the tai chi in action. It's a means of looking at the environment, in which life is seen as a kind of dance, an interplay of opposites. When this is reflected in physical movement, the result is the exercise system known as Tai Chi Chuan.

# The tai chi form

The special arrangement of movements that you will find in these pages is collectively called a 'form'. The form is made up of lots of separate movements which are eventually strung together to produce one continuous sequence lasting several minutes. The movements are always done in the same order, like the components of a specially choreographed dance. The wonderful thing about tai chi is that most of these separate movements have a Yang and a Yin aspect. So when you do tai chi you are also participating in the interplay of opposites: harmonising yourself over and over again with the cyclic forces of nature. The individual 'tao' then becomes connected to the greater, universal Tao. Tai chi is a celebration of nature and of your place within it.

# Origins of tai chi

There have been, and still are, many different kinds of tai chi, the origins going back very far indeed and, inevitably, cloaked in their fair share of mystery and legend. For example, Huang Ti, the legendary Yellow Emperor of China, was said to have practised special exercises for maintaining health, based on the observation of animals, as long ago as 2700 BC. This is the earliest reference we have to anything like tai chi. But, as with acupuncture and the many other branches of medicine and self-culture begun by the Chinese, activities of this kind probably have their origin in the days before recorded history. Incidentally Huang Ti was said to have reigned for a hundred years and to have had over a hundred wives, so he must have been doing *something* right!

Around the thirteenth century, these exercises seem to have joined forces with the martial arts, or were at least developed by them to great effect. The martial arts in China were at that time being practised to a very high standard by the Ch'an (Zen) Buddhist monks. And although no one really knows for sure how the process took place, the combination of all these diverse strands of thought and action eventually gave birth to the practice of Tai Chi Chuan (the great way or system of tai chi) as we know it today.

For all the historical confusion surrounding the subject, this has not in any way discouraged the spread of numerous stories concerning the origin of tai chi. One of the most interesting of these relates to the illusive 'founder' of the art, Chang San-feng, a Taoist priest – *illusive* because he is reported as having lived in various places at various times, in some instances a few centuries apart!

The legend has it that one evening he had a particularly vivid dream in which he saw a great bird – a crane – and a snake engaged in combat over a morsel of food. Neither creature seemed to be able to overcome the other. Each time the snake attempted to sink his fangs into the crane, the

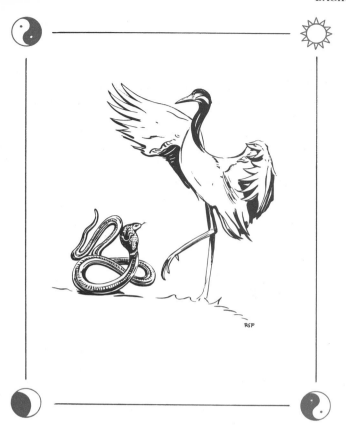

bird would gracefully side-step and enfold the creature in its powerful wing and sweep it away. Each time the crane tried to crush the snake or pierce it with its sharp beak, the snake would recoil and twist, often launching a counter-attack of its own. The beauty and grace of this contest impressed Chang greatly. The next night he had the same dream. Once more, the crane would come down from the heavens and the snake up from the earth and the contest would begin again.

The Yang and Yin imagery here is very powerful and symbolic of an eternal contest, the eternal state of dynamic balance in nature, exemplified in the Tai Chi T'u.

It is probably because of stories of this kind, and the alliance with the fighting monks of medieval China, that tai chi often appears somewhat martial in character when compared to the numerous comparatively passive chi-generating exercises from which it originally sprang. There is a common energy pattern used both for health and for martial skills, and what is good for one is invariably good for the other. Thus, these two often quite disparate applications of tai chi in the modern world still exist quite happily side by side.

The kind of tai chi we will be devoting ourselves to in this book is a somewhat more recent variation on this great tradition, called the Yang style. Although itself a development based on a long tradition of tai chi technique, this Yang style emerged as recently as the nineteenth century. Its founder was Lu Chuan Yang who lived from 1799 to 1872. His grandson, Cheng Fu Yang, taught tai chi into the twentieth century and it was one of his pupils, Cheng Man Ching, who most helped to spread tai chi in the West – basically by shortening the form into a concise eight-minute sequence. This is called, naturally enough, the 'short Yang form' and is the form featured in this book.

# How long does it take to learn?

I once heard a fellow student ask the question in a tai chi class 'How long does it take?'. The reply was, 'Well, how long have you got?', implying that, in a sense, you never really reach the end of the learning process. Nevertheless, it was a reasonable question and if it could possibly be modified to something like, 'How long will it take before I can do the form all the way through and gain some benefits from it?', the answer would probably be less ambiguous. But it still depends on how much you are prepared to work at it. There are no short cuts or fast results with tai chi. It takes around six months to learn the form adequately and a lifetime to master it. As you learn, it is essential to practise every day for around ten minutes, adding newly learned movements each time. Then, once you have learned the form, you *still* keep on working at it every day. Ultimately, you will be spending at least 15–20 minutes daily on your tai chi studies, since these might eventually also include some reading, meditation and breathing exercises.

The best time to do tai chi is in the morning or evening, when the forces of Yang and Yin are most harmonised (sunrise and sunset). Outdoors is best, for there you will find an abundance of natural energy. Traditionally, tai chi is done beneath trees or near water. But any time and anywhere is better than never. The more you work at it, the quicker you will learn – simple as that.

# What are the benefits?

Numerous independent scientific studies, both in the West and in China and Japan, have proved beyond any shadow of a doubt the enormous benefits that tai chi and its related disciplines of chi kung (additional breathing techniques that we will be looking at later) can bring in terms of good health, recovery from illness and the strengthening of the immune system.

Of course, we all know that exercise helps us to keep fit and therefore to stay well. This is because exercise helps to maintain the heart and lungs and so improve the circulation. Tai chi, however, goes far beyond this, since it enhances the health and performance of all the organs and systems of the body. Tai chi also works on a deep emotional level as well.

It puts us in touch with our body's needs, strengthening the mind, calming the emotions and releasing considerable personal creativity in the process. It helps us to cope with stress and to find solutions to problems more easily.

All this takes time to cultivate, of course. But here are some of the benefits that should come to you fairly soon, providing you really do practise every day. You will start to notice an overall improvement in balance after just a few weeks so that you feel stronger and firmer on your feet. You will become more relaxed, especially after doing the form; more aware and content. Your circulation will improve, your joints become more mobile and, as long as you take care of yourself and avoid the obvious drawbacks of junk food, cigarettes and other stimulants, your overall state of health will strengthen.

# *The nature of chi*

Translations into English of the word 'chi', or 'qi' as it is sometimes written, are many and varied. The nearest term we have for chi in our own language is probably 'life force' or 'vital energy'. Those already practising yoga will be familiar with this concept as 'prana'.

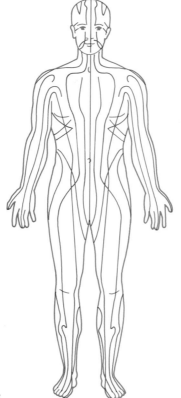

*Fig. 2   The energy channels*

We store chi in our bodies. Chi is to be found in the lines of force, or 'meridians' as they are called, which circulate through the body and which are used in oriental medicine to balance the internal energies and so maintain health. This is why a doctor specialising in acupuncture or shiatsu can improve, say, the state of your lungs by stimulating the surface of the body with small needles or finger pressure. When we practise tai chi, we are not only absorbing this vital energy through our breathing but are also setting the chi in motion around our bodies.

The body is a wonderful self-regulating system. It uses the vital energy where and when it needs it. You simply set the chi in motion; the body takes care of the rest. Figure 2 gives a representation of the superficial energetic pattern of the body. There are many deeper channels, supporting these.

Recent scientific investigation has located the distribution of chi in the human body and has found this to correspond closely to the old medical charts of the Chinese acupuncture system – mapped out all those centuries ago by the brilliant doctors and physicians of those times. It has been found that each acu-point has a lower electrical resistance than the surrounding tissues; and so also with the acupuncture channels, along which all these points are ranged – thereby validating the entire basis of oriental medicine which, naturally, assumes the existence of chi as a first principle.

For centuries in the East, such knowledge had been in broad circulation, of course, and today, those of us working in the field of oriental medicine need no proof of the existence of the body's subtle energetic system, since we can feel it for ourselves during treatment. But it is good to know that anybody embarking on a course of tai chi study, or any related system of energetic body work, can do so today confident that they are dealing with very real forces that work deep within the human body, sustaining it and nourishing it, throughout its life.

Incidentally, outside the body, science has also located something akin to chi in the electrical field of the atmosphere. There are certain electrically charged particles in the atmosphere, positive and negative ions in the air we breathe. The positive ions are associated with dust and pollution and are to be found mostly in cities, while the negative ions are in abundance in clean, moist air, in sunlight or by the sea. Thus, as we all know, housework and traffic jams are debilitating, but fresh air and trips to the seaside are invigorating. This is why tai chi places such emphasis on the breath and on practising outdoors wherever possible.

Whatever way you look at it, tai chi has got to be good news, and in the next chapter we will look at how to begin working on the form and getting in touch with these internal energies through the tai chi movements themselves.

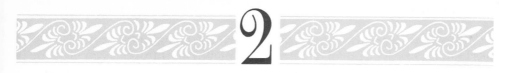

# 2

# *GENTLY DOES IT*

There is hardly anything in life that cannot benefit from being done slowly. This is certainly true for tai chi – the movements are celebrated for their graceful, gentle quality, like a floating cloud or running stream.

During the early days of training, however, most students want to perform the movements fairly rapidly and there are two reasons for this. Firstly, human beings are impatient creatures. The more hectic and stressful the lifestyle, the more difficult it is to slow down and do anything in a relaxed fashion.

Secondly, most of us tend to move in a rather unbalanced, haphazard fashion most of the time. When walking, for instance – and no matter how well co-ordinated and confident we might feel – we tend rather to 'fall' into each step instead of placing the feet in a controlled way. This is natural enough for anyone wanting to get from A to B quickly, but it's not what we're looking for in tai chi. Those who spend a little time practising the form, however, soon learn to control their movements and direct them precisely. This in turn draws the body and mind into a state of relaxation and harmony.

Of course it isn't easy at first. Patience and self-discipline need to be cultivated, qualities that you will develop through regular practice and which will set a pattern for attaining many other kinds of self-control, helping you to focus your mind, cultivate detachment and achieve results more easily through enhanced levels of concentration.

As well as developing balance and physical stability, or what is called 'rooting', the slowness of the tai chi movements also concentrates and generates the vital energy of the body, bathing all the organs in lifegiving chi. The slow pace also serves to work thoroughly many of the muscles of the body (in tai chi, particularly the legs) and therefore helps to maintain a healthy circulation.

## *How fast? How slow?*

So exactly how slowly should we be moving in tai chi? It may come as a surprise to those just starting out, but there are no hard and fast rules for this. The answer is different for each person and depends on how thoroughly you are able to relax and also, later on, upon the natural rhythm of your breathing.

These days, the short Yang form described in Chapters 4 and 5 normally takes around eight minutes to perform, though it can be done faster if you wish – and it certainly can, and often is, done slower. It could be argued that there has recently been a marked trend, especially here in the West, to slow the whole thing down. When western folk first see tai chi, their immediate observation is 'Oh, look – how slow it all is!' As a consequence, when they take it up they turn it into something even slower! In particular, this tendency grew apace during the 1960s, when it was considered really 'cool' to do tai chi in a kind of trancelike mood.

Well, there is nothing wrong with feeling calm during your tai chi. You *should* feel calm. But you should also be alert and aware and not moving so slowly that you become tense and impatient with yourself. Cheng Man Ching – who, after all, originated the very sequence we are studying here – once wrote that he created the short form because he couldn't spend a lot of time each day performing the traditional long form. His own shortened version, he stated, could be got through in just four minutes! That suited him.

Viewed in this light, our modern eight-minute sequence might seem rather self-indulgent but the fact of the matter is, providing your limbs are relaxed and you feel the chi flowing, it doesn't matter a jot how fast or how slow you do it. The main thing is that you *do it* – and enjoy the experience.

# *Breathing made visible*

The first thing we do when we come into this world is breathe. And when we cease to be, so also do we cease to breathe. We can do without food for weeks, without liquids for days, but most of us would be hard pressed to do without air for more than a few minutes and it is little wonder that people the world over have always thought of the breath as containing the very essence and spirit of life.

When going through the tai chi form, the breath should be evenly distributed between the contracting and the expanding movements. These movements are actually timed to the breathing: in other words, gathering in during each inhalation and projecting out with the natural exhalation that follows. This is important since the energy, both muscular and vital energy, moves better when exhaling, which is why weightlifters breathe out suddenly during the main lift and why those doing karate cry out during their punches or kicks. This serves to expel the air efficiently and move the chi at exactly the right moment. In tai chi we remain silent, of course, but we should still always be exhaling gently during the projecting movements of the form – i.e. with movements such as Push (page 27) or Press (page 26).

Naturally, then, we would want to *inhale* in between these projecting movements – for example, the movements such as Rollback (page 25) or the Pull (page 32). However, most parts of the form that feature inbreathing are not provided with names. Instead, the inbreath is usually viewed as a prelude to each named movement. Therefore, an inbreath precedes the Ward Off (page 23), Push (page 27) and so on.

## Finding your rhythm

Try this brief experiment and with a quick bit of arithmetic, you should be able to settle on a rhythm and a pace that is right for you.

Firstly, take a moment to relax; walk around a bit and see how slowly you can breathe without feeling agitated or short of wind. How often – ten times a minute? Twelve times a minute? There are precisely 80 cycles of breathing in the form shown in this book so if you do an eight-minute form, this works out at ten breaths per minute, or one typical tai chi movement every five to six seconds. If this feels too slow for you right now, don't worry. Speed it up! A faster, seven-minute form lets you take about 12 breaths a minute, or one cycle every four to five seconds.

Whatever pace you settle on, the main thing is to keep in synchronisation with the breathing instructions accompanying the illustrations and to breathe naturally and gently at a calm, regular pace all the way through. Above all, *don't force it*! Find your own speed and don't take the above guidelines so literally that you have to use your stopwatch. There is no such thing as a Tai Chi Inspector who is going to pop out of the bushes and upbraid you for doing your form in five minutes instead of 15. Do what comes naturally and you'll be fine.

I once had a student who wanted to learn tai chi. When I asked him whether he did any kind of exercise already, he replied, 'No, but I always go out into the garden every morning and do about ten minutes of deep breathing'.

'Fine,' I answered. 'You are already half-way towards doing tai chi! All you need now is to add some body movement, shaped around the breathing, and you're there!'

Tai chi is *breathing made visible*. The breath is the source and the destination of all your tai chi studies. This is why it is sometimes referred to as a 'moving meditation' – since all forms of meditation require a quietening of the mind through regular, rhythmic breathing. A useful and pleasing metaphor is to think of the in and outbreaths as solar and lunar respectively. Tai Yang is actually a Chinese term for the Sun (the Great Light), while Tai Yin is the Moon (the Great Dark). You will encounter these solar and lunar principles more and more as you progress with your tai chi studies. Most worthwhile things in life have a mystical dimension and tai chi is certainly no exception. And it is largely through the contemplation and realisation of the harmony between Yang and Yin that such experiences can be attained.

66 *There is an inward centre in ourselves where truth abides in fullness.* 99

Robert Browning

# Practice, practice, practice

For practice it is best to have a routine of some kind, i.e. the same time every day if you can. The most favourable times are considered to be early in the morning or in the evening, but any time will do, providing you can spend at least ten minutes each session. In China and other eastern countries, people from all walks of life are to be found every morning in the parks and open spaces, working on their exercises, including tai chi. It is part of their daily routine and sets them up for the rigours of what is to come. Indeed, most teachers of tai chi will tell you that it is essential to practise every day and preferably a couple of times every day if you can. But for someone just starting out you can reduce this to once daily.

And don't feel that you have to be up at the crack of dawn for this. That's fine for some but if you lead a complex life, working an eight-hour day, commuting, cooking meals, putting the children to bed and doing housework each evening as well, you are probably entitled *not* to get up at the crack of dawn. Does that mean that you cannot benefit from tai chi? Of course not. Simply find a convenient space in your daily routine; be happy with the situation and try to stick with it.

Being properly prepared for practice is always a good idea and the wearing of loose, comfortable clothing and sensible footwear is essential. Make sure you are reasonably calm and collected before you approach your tai chi sessions. Never rush into the movements with haste or with reluctance – that would only be a waste of time. Likewise, never do tai chi when you have just eaten or if you are angry or upset over anything. If necessary, sit quietly for a moment and put the mind at rest before beginning. You owe that to yourself.

You should also make sure you have a peaceful location; either a quiet, uncluttered room where you will not be disturbed or, best of all, outdoors. If necessary, make it clear to your family that you will be setting aside ten or 15 minutes for yourself each day. This is a time *just for you* and should not involve others in any sense. Children and pets are particularly uncooperative about anyone doing tai chi in their midst. There is no need to be mysterious or secretive about your tai chi studies. Just explain your intentions and what is required and that way your desire for privacy will usually be respected. Finally, don't forget to take the phone off the hook!

# Getting started

The tai chi form should always be preceded by a brief warm-up session, particularly in cold weather. That way the body gets the maximum benefit from the form. Any kind of gentle exercise will do for warming up, although there are numerous Chinese-style routines that can be used and which you will acquire in abundance should you ever attend formal classes in tai chi. What is important, however, is that you gently stretch the limbs and loosen the joints. Don't overdo this, though. Warming up should never be so lengthy as to leave you with no time or energy for anything else. Keep it simple.

Here are some suggestions:

**1** Stand with feet shoulder width apart, bend the knees a little, relax the shoulders and slowly allow your arms to swing back and forth together at your side. Do this for a while and then pick up an imaginary ball between your hands and throw it up into the air. Relax the neck muscles as you do this and allow the spine to gently stretch back. Then return to your rocking (Fig. 3).

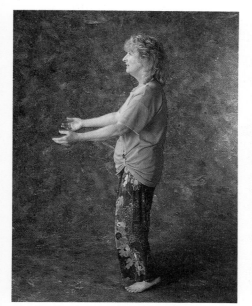 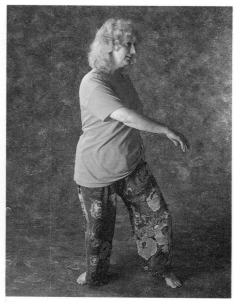

*Fig. 3    Rocking exercise*              *Fig. 4    Twisting exercise*

**2** Spread the feet a little further apart and then twist the body from side to side, moving from the waist and allowing your arms to flop around as you turn: very loose, like a rag doll. As you twist to the side, raise the opposite heel slightly. Always aim to keep the knees apart, as if seated upon a nice plump horse; do not let the knees drift in towards each other as you turn. Let the arms 'lengthen'. Relax the spine, chest, neck and shoulders (Fig. 4).

> **66** *The theory and function of Tai Chi principles are found everywhere.* **99**
>
> Cheng Man Ch'ing

**3**  With your feet again shoulder width apart, extend the arms in front of you and simply rotate the wrists slowly, several times in each direction. Squeeze your hands into fists, open them up, fingers wide apart, and then shake – shake the whole hand loosely and allow the shaking to extend right up the arms so that the wrists, elbows and even perhaps the shoulders start to loosen also.

**4**  Rotate the ankles in a similar fashion (one at a time, of course). Stretch out the toes and then shake or kick – again allowing the sensation to extend upwards, in this case to the knees and maybe even the hips if you can.

**5**  Rotate the neck – gently please – easing away any tightness you might feel. Make sure your hands are not screwed up into fists as you do this. Remember, the nerves and blood vessels of the arm originate in the neck and shoulders so relax them. Relax the arms and fingers. You can even bend the knees a little too.

**6**  Placing the feet as wide apart as you can, squat down on one foot, getting a progressive stretch along the inside of one leg (Fig. 5). Then change sides and stretch along the other leg. Experiment with different ways in which you can use this kind of movement to stretch different parts of the leg.

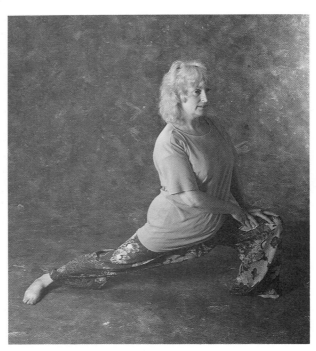

*Fig. 5*
*Leg stretches*

**7**  Circle the arms up and slowly around, loosening the shoulders. Rotate them both together or alternately, like swimming backstroke and crawl. Shake out the arms again when you have done.

And now you are ready for your tai chi form.

# 3

# TIPS AND SUGGESTIONS

## Do's and don'ts

The tai chi form you are about to learn comes in two parts. The next chapter sets out the first part and if you are a complete newcomer, you should be aiming to learn this first. Many people are satisfied with doing just Part One – a brief, two-minute sequence. They repeat this several times through and arguably derive just as many benefits in terms of health as those who do the whole form. There is no disgrace, therefore, if this is as far as you wish to go and if you can go through it a few times every day, you will already be making great strides towards good health and a relaxed mind.

Even when you graduate to Part Two, always learn each movement *thoroughly* before going on. Remember, you are putting together a string of pearls here and each one must be added on carefully before the next. This will not only ensure that you remember what you have learnt, but that you will be able to call upon past movements whenever they need to be repeated, as they often are, later in the sequence. Take a day to learn each movement and after a few months you will have the whole thing.

A common question at this stage is, 'Can tai chi be combined with other forms of exercise or sport?'. The answer is, quite simply, 'Yes'. Tai chi will help improve your skills in any sport or recreational activity. In my experience it blends particularly well with the gentle stretching exercises of yoga and in fact there is a whole branch of taoist yoga very similar to the classical Indian hatha yoga that most people are familiar with. So you don't have to give anything up. As long as you find time for practice, you will succeed. A sensible diet, free of junk food, will speed your progress, as will the use of therapies, such as shiatsu or acupuncture, which help to maintain health and vitality. These should be undertaken regularly, as a matter of course, and not just in times of illness.

Before you embark on the instruction section, it would be helpful to understand a few basic principles of tai chi movement and also to become familiar with the basic stances and methods of getting around.

> **66** *You must wave the arm and let the palm move against the wind, feeling the air as if it were water.* **99**
>
> Cheng Man Ch'ing

# *Posture*

## Relax the shoulders

Always be aware of what is happening in your shoulders and try to let them relax as much as possible. When raising the arms, for instance, try not to tense the muscles of the neck. Whenever the arms are extended out in front of you, keep them low.

## Never lock the elbows or knees

By locking, I mean straightening the arms or legs completely, so the joints are stiff. This inhibits the circulation of blood and chi and only serves to create tension in the whole of the body.

## Keep a low centre of gravity

Imagine your weight and your breath becoming concentrated in your abdomen area. Be aware of your body's centre, which in tai chi is considered to be just beneath the navel and slightly inwards towards the spine – the 'Tan Tien', as it is called. Keep your knees soft and flexible throughout and think of being close to the ground, well rooted and stealth-like.

## Allow the spine to hang loose

At all times, imagine you are being suspended from above by – traditionally, it is said – a golden thread, attached to the top of your head.

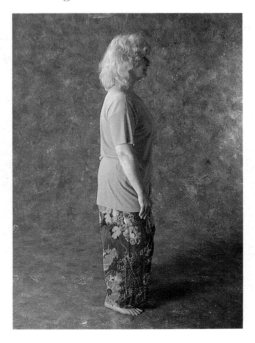

*Fig. 6   Posture*

The spine 'hangs', therefore, like a plumb line, totally vertical and relaxed. To assist this process, tuck in your backside by raising the pelvic bones and draw back the chin (Fig. 6). Make sure you do this in a relaxed fashion – no tension, please. Standing like this – let alone moving like it – is an art that has to be cultivated so be patient; be mindful of it and it will eventually happen.

# Basic stances

## The wide 70/30 stance

The width between the feet in the majority of stances is approximately the distance between your shoulders from tip to tip – a measurement to be known as 'shoulder width' from here on. It is important to remember that even if you have one foot way ahead of the other, they both remain on lines that would run back directly to beneath your shoulders. It may be helpful to think of yourself standing on tram lines (Fig. 7). A rather small tram, admittedly, but the principle is sound. In this stance, you will either have 70% of your weight forward in the leading leg or 70% behind in the rear leg – hence the term 70/30 stance. Sometimes, as you go from one movement to the next, this ratio of weight alternates between the two legs without moving the feet. The foot diagrams accompanying each photograph in the instruction section will help you to achieve the correct distribution.

*Note:* except when you are transferring from one position to another, the front knee never extends beyond the tip of the foot (Fig. 8).

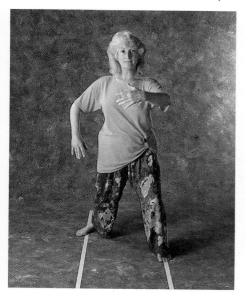

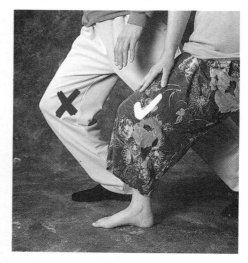

*Fig. 7    Wide stance*

*Fig. 8    Knee over toes*

## The narrow heel stance

In this position, most of your weight settles in the back foot, allowing just the front heel to make contact with the ground. In this, and the narrow toe stance mentioned next, the front foot is more or less in a line ahead of the back heel – the ratio of weight being around 90% back foot, 10% front. When moving into a narrow stance it is helpful, and indeed recommended, to turn in the foot a little at the very start, by pivoting on the heel. This is not, incidentally, strictly the way Cheng Man Ching taught it but is rather more in keeping with the traditional Yang style that preceded his own. This way is good for us, however, since it assists in relieving any tension felt in the knee when maintaining a narrow stance for any length of time.

## The narrow toe stance

This is identical to the previous posture, only it is the toes of the leading foot which just lightly make contact with the ground. Again, the ratio is around 90/10 – and again, the back foot is adjusted before the movement to ensure that the back knee remains free of tension.

# Getting about

## Always sink into the substantial leg before stepping

As the tai chi steps are always slow, it is important to feel well balanced in what is called the 'substantial' leg – the one that bears your weight. So before stepping, bend the knee and always sink your weight into the substantial leg, and only slowly raise the other foot, testing your balance all the while. That way you will be able to raise the foot and place it down wherever you want it, gently and under control. You should never lunge or stumble into a movement.

## Step forward heel first; step back toes first

This is self-explanatory. Most of your steps are forward ones, in fact, but when you do them, make sure it is your heel and not any other part of your foot that first makes contact with the ground. That way the knee will bend easily and naturally, permitting you to flatten the rest of the foot onto the ground slowly. Conversely, if you need to step backwards or put the foot down behind, do so by making contact with the toes first.

## Move from the centre

Often in tai chi it looks as if the arms are very active, but in fact it is the legs, the waist and the body which are doing most of the work. This is highly characteristic of most tai chi technique. The movement begins from the centre, the Tan Tien mentioned above. Be aware of this place and allow it to guide your movements like a beam of light. Keep those arms and shoulders relaxed!

## Adjust the back foot after stepping

Following most forward steps into a wide 70/30 stance, you will feel the need to pivot slightly on your back heel to find a comfortable position and to take any tension out of your knee.

*Note:* if you end up moving on your back toes instead and your back hip feels all locked up and tense, then you have most probably not stepped into a wide enough stance. Remember the tram lines: shoulder width apart.

## Keep the knee over the substantial foot

Try not to let your knee drift inside the substantial foot (Fig. 9 shows the right and the wrong way of doing this). If it keeps wanting to do this, you may possibly have an energy imbalance in the acu-channels that run on the inside or outside of the leg. Shiatsu treatment is recommended to alleviate this.

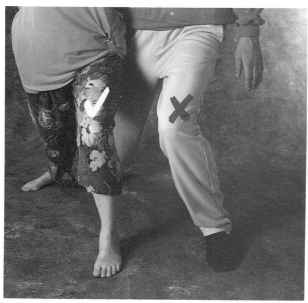

*Fig. 9   Knee drifting inside substantial foot*

## Use your imagination

Always endeavour to project mental energy into the actions. When a hand extends outwards, for example, let the energy go with it – *think* it outwards. Also, tai chi is often best learned with the aid of imagery, some of which may sound rather bizarre at first. Stroking the pony's nose or holding a ball or throwing your fist – it may all seem a bit strange but you will find this sort of thing helpful during the early stages of learning. As you become more proficient you will, of course, be able to discard the images altogether and enjoy the beauty of the movements themselves.

## Continuous movement

Although the form is made up of separate pieces, it should be executed as one continuous, flowing sequence. Do not stop at any point. Let the hands and arms 'float' gently from one movement into the next, without pause.

## Directions in the foot diagrams

At the start of the form, you face 'south' – the favourite and most auspicious direction in Chinese popular culture. East is therefore on your left-hand side, west on your right. It is not necessary, of course, to line up with the actual compass direction of south, but simply decide on a point of reference before you start and call it 'south'. These imaginary cardinal points are very helpful for the purposes of conveying information from teacher to student – as will become obvious as you start to learn.

That's it! All rather a lot to take in, especially as you are probably raring to go and get on with learning the form itself. However, you will benefit from referring back to these pages from time to time, especially if things aren't quite working out the way you expected. If you feel uncomfortable at any time, check the points above to find out why.

> **66** *The hands sweep upwards and downward in a diagonal motion, resembling the flying pattern of a bird winging low over the banks of a river.* **99**
>
> Da Liu, referring to Diagonal (or Slant) Flying

# 4

# THE FORM – PART ONE

> 66 *He who pursues Tao will decrease every day. He will decrease and continue to decrease, 'til he comes to non-action. By non-action everything can be done.* 99
>
> Tao Te Ching

# *Step-by-step instructions*

## Opening (Photos 1–6)

1   Stand facing south, feet together, toes pointing out and the heels not quite touching. Take a moment to experience how the body feels. Tuck in the base of the spine and relax the shoulders and fingers. Make space under your arms, as if you have a large egg under each armpit. Breathe in gently and begin.

*Note:* make sure your spine is vertical, as if suspended from above, as illustrated on page 14.

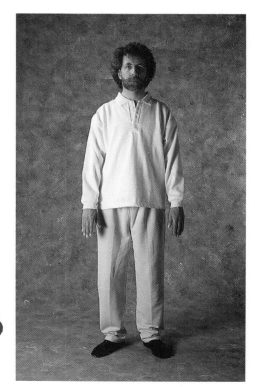

*1   OPENING*
*Inbreath*

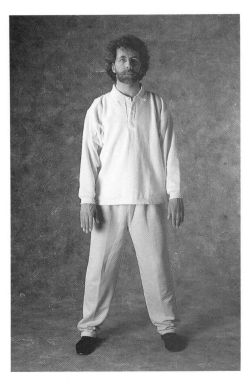

2   Sink onto the right foot. Raise the left foot and place it down to the east, shoulder width from your right, the toes pointing south. Adjust your right foot so that it also points south. The feet are parallel, therefore, and the weight evenly distributed. The foot diagram here shows the new rectangle on which you should be standing (solid line) as well as the location of the previous rectangle (dotted line). This technique will be adopted occasionally in these pages to enable you to see major changes in position more clearly.

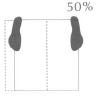

50%

*2   OPENING*
*Outbreath*

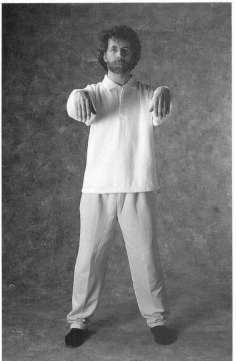

3   With wrists relaxed and fingers pointing slightly downwards, allow your arms to rise to about chest height, the forearms parallel with the ground. Let the arms 'float' upwards – though only as far as you can comfortably go. The shoulders should remain still when the arms rise – one of the ways in which tai chi teaches us to relax and, in time, to eliminate tension from that area altogether. The neck and shoulders are, of course, a common place for tension and pain to gather. Keep them relaxed!

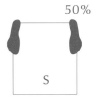

50%

S

*3   OPENING*
*Inbreath*

4   As your breathe out, very slowly raise and straighten your fingers so that the tips are pointing south. Think, also, of the wrists dropping as well as the fingers straightening. Do this without tension. Monitor the stiffness or otherwise of your finger joints during this exercise. How slowly can you move them without them shaking or tightening up? The more relaxed you can make your hands, the better will be the blood supply to the joints.

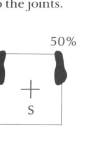

**50%**

**4   OPENING**
*Outbreath*

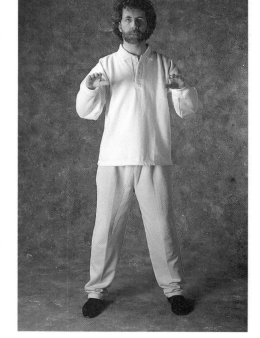

5   Draw the elbows back. Try to keep your arms away from your sides. Look at the illustration closely. See how much space there is between the elbows and the sides. Be aware, also, of the space behind, between your shoulder blades. Make sure that, in drawing the elbows back, you do not create tension in this place. Bring the elbows back only as far as is comfortable.

**50%**

**5   OPENING**
*Inbreath*

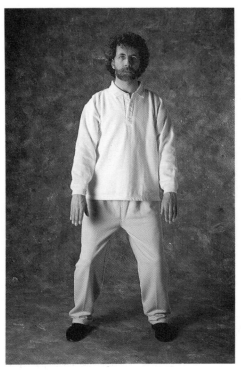

6 Lower your arms slowly to your sides and let your weight sink. Try to imagine roots going down into the ground from your feet. Relax the shoulders, relax the fingers and let the knees bend a little too. Try to feel a connection with the ground beneath you, but at the same time continue to imagine your body suspended – traditionally described as a 'golden thread' attached to the top of the head and going right up into the sky.

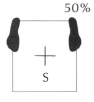

50%

*6   OPENING*
*Outbreath*

## Turn Right (Photos 7–8)

7 Sink onto the left foot and turn your waist slowly to the west by pivoting on your right heel. Do not raise the right heel – this is not a step, just a turn. Simultaneously, raise the right arm to a near vertical position but with the wrist loose, palm down. The left hand, meanwhile, rises as well – palm up – to 'cup' the right elbow. The term 'cupping the elbow' should not be taken too literally. There is plenty of space between your upturned palm and the elbow, and the palm is also not directly beneath it. Think of holding a large ball and try to get the movements of the waist and the arms to flow smoothly together.

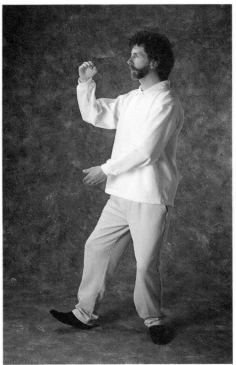

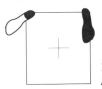

90%

*7   TURN RIGHT*
*Inbreath*

8    Allow the right foot to go flat down
and shift your weight onto it, so that
the knee goes just over the tip of your
toes as you look down. Your right
hand is at about chin height, your eyes
looking over it towards an imaginary
distant horizon. Try to feel the ball,
the chi connection, between your
palms. Keep the back straight.

*Note:* at first, as you learn this
movement, you will need to
concentrate on the hands and feet
separately, but it does not take long
before the whole thing starts to flow.
Keep trying, until all of the body feels
co-ordinated.

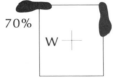

*8    TURN RIGHT*
*Outbreath*

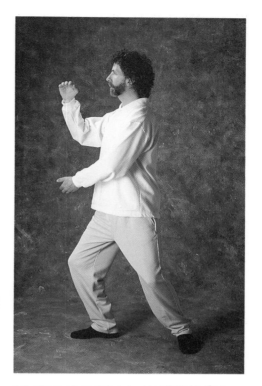

# Ward Off Left (Photos 9–10)

9    Here we meet with the first step
into a wide 70/30 stance. Sink onto
your right foot and raise your left heel,
preparing to step southwards with
your left leg. Uncurl the right hand
slighly, to show your palm to the south
before you go. Try to retain the feeling
of the palms being in communication
with one another. Even though you
have let go of the ball now, imagine it is
somehow still attracted to your hands.

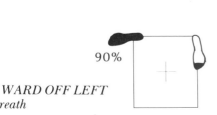

*9    WARD OFF LEFT*
*Inbreath*

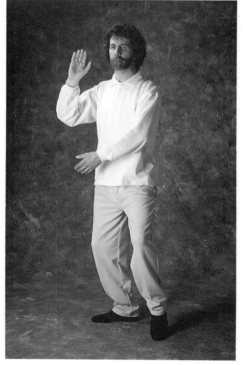

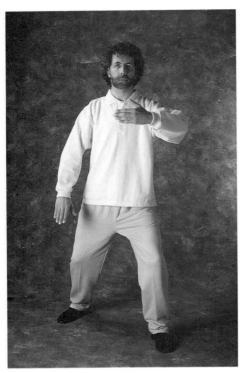

10    Step out south with your left heel and bend the knee. Simultaneously, raise the left arm into a horizontal position in front of your chest, palm in, and drop your right arm to your side. The surfaces of the two palms seem to figuratively 'stroke' each other at a distance as they go, one rising, one falling. If you have made a proper job of this, your head, hips and shoulders should all be facing south, nicely squared up. If this is not the case, and if you feel uncomfortably twisted, refer to Chapter 3 for help and try again.

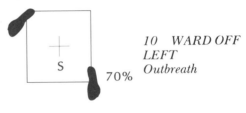

70%

*10   WARD OFF LEFT*
*Outbreath*

## Grasp Bird's Tail (Photos 11–12)

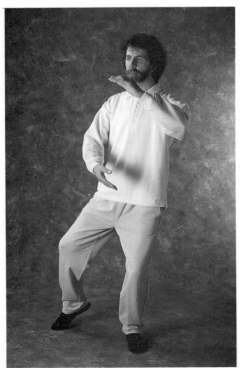

11    Sink onto your left foot and raise your right heel. At the same time allow your centre to turn slightly to your left and get your right hand to swoop around with it to 'pick up a ball' – about the size of the a large beach ball – with the left hand on top, right hand underneath.

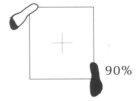

90%

*11   GRASP BIRD'S TAIL*
*Inbreath*

12   Turn your waist and step to the west with your right heel. Bend the right knee and bring 70% of your weight forward. Carry the ball with you, only imagine it getting smaller, so that your right hand finishes up at the level of your chest, the arm slanting upwards somewhat and a little out to the side, the fingers of your left hand, meanwhile, pointing towards your right palm. Finally, adjust the left foot to a comfortable position by pivoting on the heel. Your head, hips and shoulders face due west – right knee over right toes. Do not overstretch. Keep the arms in a rounded, embracing kind of aspect rather than thrusting them too far ahead.

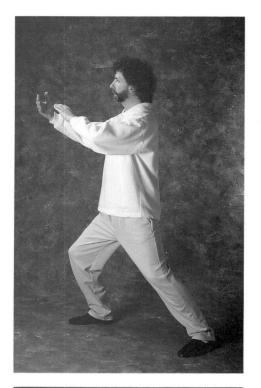

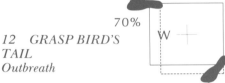

*12   GRASP BIRD'S TAIL*
*Outbreath*

## Rollback (Photo 13)

13   The name of this movement is very descriptive. What happens is that you roll your hands, so that for a moment your left palm is looking up, your right looking down. Then, without moving your feet or raising your toes, you shift your weight back onto your left leg. At the same time, allow the left hand to 'cup' the right elbow – a little like you did earlier with Turn Right, but this time with the right fingers pointing upwards, palm facing south. During his movement, your centre turns very slightly to your right.

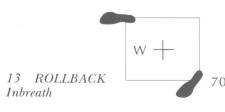

*13   ROLLBACK*
*Inbreath*

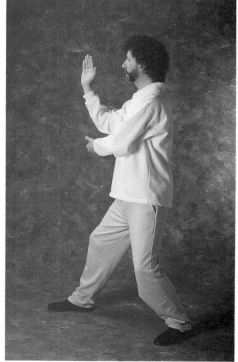

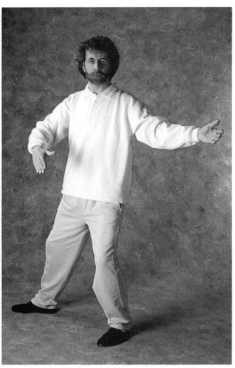

## Press (Photos 14–15)

14   Without moving your feet, turn the waist counter-clockwise, towards the south. Open up the left shoulder and circle back with your left hand, palm up. At the same time, fold your right forearm down to a near horizontal position across your centre, palm down. Try to get a feeling for the hands moving together, even though they are quite a distance from each other, moving round with your centre.

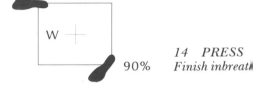

90%

*14   PRESS*
*Finish inbreath*

15   As you start to exhale, bring the weight forward once again into your right foot. Draw your left hand forwards and around to your middle as the waist itself rotates back towards the west. Then bring your palms together at about chest height in front of you, the heels of the palms themselves just lightly making contact. You are looking at the palm of your right hand and the back of your left hand, therefore, hips and shoulders facing west, right knee over right toes.

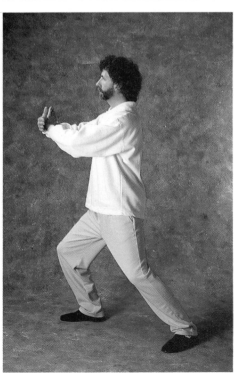

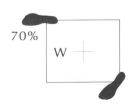

70%

*15   PRESS*
*Outbreath*

# Separate Hands and Push (Photos 16–17)

16   Again, the name given to this movement is very descriptive. What you do is simply separate your hands in a little swimming motion in front of your chest, palms down, and then sit back once again onto your rear leg. Do it slowly, trailing your right thumb across beneath your left palm as you separate the hands, and then try to imagine the lung energies in your chest as you breathe in. Keep your elbows away from your sides to encourage the breathing process.

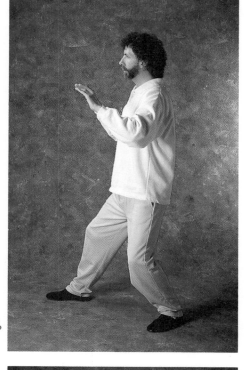

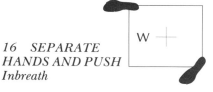

*16   SEPARATE HANDS AND PUSH*
*Inbreath*

70%

17   Bring the weight forward once again, right knee over right toes, and turn the palms out to create the effect of pushing forward at chest height. Don't feel that you need to thrust your arms forward to do this. You only need to turn the palms out and extend the arms a tiny bit, the rest being achieved by the forward movement of your body, created essentially from the bending of the right knee. Make sure you do not lean forward.

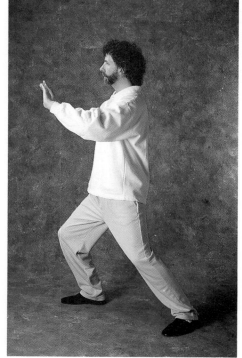

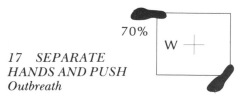

70%

*17   SEPARATE HANDS AND PUSH*
*Outbreath*

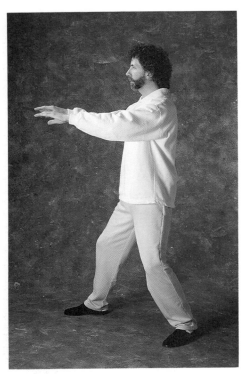

# Single Whip (Photos 18–23)

18   One of the more intricate movements of the tai chi form now follows. Firstly, sit back once again on the rear leg and turn your palms down. If you keep your arms where they are they will appear to lengthen out as a consequence of shifting your weight back, as shown in the illustration. Do not lock the elbows. The arms are straight but not rigid. And of course keep the knees relaxed, too.

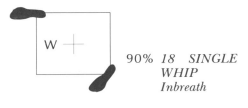

90%  *18   SINGLE WHIP Inbreath*

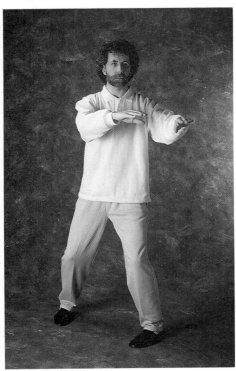

19   With most of your weight in the left foot, turn your waist counter-clockwise and pivot slowly on your right heel as you go. Your arms will naturally follow, the result being that your fingers will tend to point south-east and your feet will become slightly pigeon-toed. This may feel a little uncomfortable at first. The insides of your feet might want to curl off the ground or your knees might 'cave in'. However, because you are going to step way around to the east in a moment (see photo 23), it is a good idea to get that right foot as far around as you can now, in readiness.

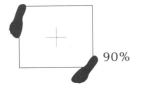

90%

*19   SINGLE WHIP Outbreath*

20   Next, transfer most of your weight back across into your right foot and allow your waist to turn again, this time slightly clockwise. Draw your right elbow across your chest and form what is called a Crane's Beak in your right hand. This is created by dropping the wrist and bunching in the fingers against the thumb – most commonly the index finger and thumb connect, as if holding a pinch of salt. The wrist relaxes into a hook shape. Also, while all this is happening, your left hand swoops down to your right hip, palm up. Imagine holding a large balloon. The fingers of the right hand hold the neck of the balloon, while the left hand supports it from underneath.

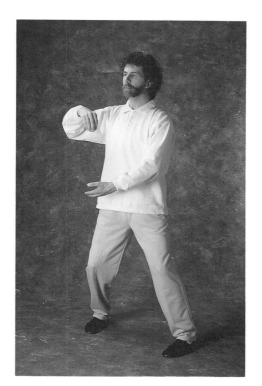

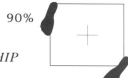

*20   SINGLE WHIP*
*Inbreath*

21   Next, pivot on your left toes, while simultaneously projecting your Crane's Beak outwards to the south-west. The right arm goes almost straight, but make sure you do not go all the way; not so straight that the arm becomes stiff. Remember, always keep the elbows and knees soft; never, ever lock them.

   *Note:* although the right arm extends outwards, much of the movement is created by rotating the waist, anti-clockwise. This, in turn, is guided or complemented by pivoting on the left toes. All parts of the body are connected in tai chi.

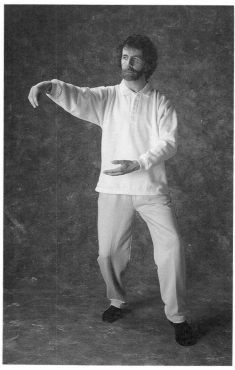

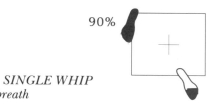

*21   SINGLE WHIP*
*Outbreath*

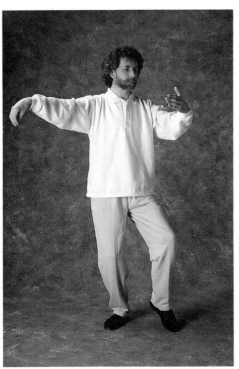

22   Sink into the right foot and raise the left foot entirely now. You are about to step around to the east and it might help you if you try drawing in your left toes towards your right heel beforehand. Start to raise the left hand and keep looking at your left palm as you begin to lift it up in front of your chest. There is a big step coming up next, so make sure you are properly balanced in your right leg before committing yourself. Remember you have lots of time – as long as it takes.

100%

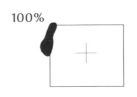

22   *SINGLE WHIP*
*Inbreath*

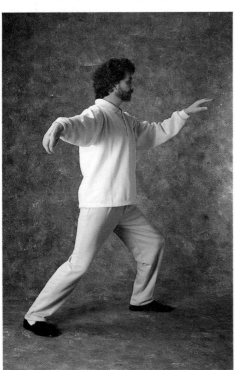

23   Now take that step around. Direct the movement from your left hip – around and slightly forward so that you can place the heel down on the far corner of a new rectangle, facing east. Keep looking at your left palm, then spiral it out and around so that the left elbow finishes in a line roughly above the left knee, the fingers pressing out to the east. Your hips and shoulders should also be facing due east, left knee over left toes. The feet are shoulder width once again – remember the tram lines?

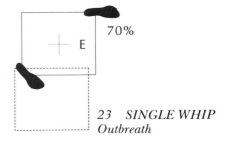

70%

E

23   *SINGLE WHIP*
*Outbreath*

# Play Guitar (Photos 24–25)

**24**   We now encounter the first narrow stance of the form. Remember, for narrow stances it is a good idea to adjust whatever foot is going to become the rear, weighted foot before you step, as clearly it would be impossible to do so once your weight is on it. So make a small adjustment now by pivoting on your left heel – not too far, but just enough to take the pressure off your knee. Then raise your right heel and pivot a little on the toes, ready to move the foot. Open your arms a little, like a bird about to flap its wings – all the while, the body is turning south and the weight transferring into your left leg.

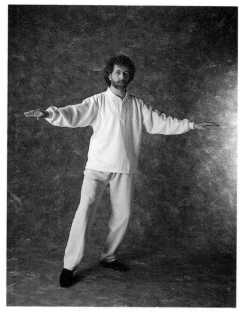

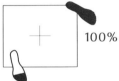

*24   PLAY GUITAR*
*Inbreath*                              100%

**25**   Draw across your right heel and place it in a narrow stance, toes pointing south and raised. The arms, meanwhile, drift in to your centre to form the typical play guitar shape – that is, in this case, with the right arm extended out ahead of you at about chest height, palm facing east, and the left arm a little nearer to you, the palm 'looking' at the inside of your right forearm. Keep the hands open, as if you are holding a big fat stick in front of you. In other words, try to sense the chi between your arms.

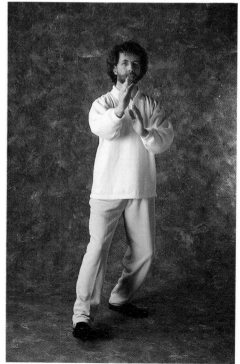

90%

*25   PLAY GUITAR*
*Outbreath*

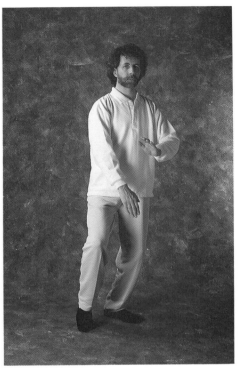

# Pull and Step with Shoulder (Photos 26–27)

26 Draw your right foot in closer to your left, the toes only in contact with the ground. At the same time lower the arms, so that your right arm hangs almost vertical at the centre. Still try to imagine there is a chi connection between your arms and hands so that they move together purposefully. This is a very Yin stance and is about as close as the feet ever get to each other in the tai chi form.

100%

*26 PULL AND STEP WITH SHOULDER*
*Inbreath*

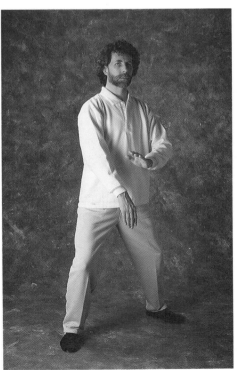

27 Step out wide with your right heel, placing the foot down, toes pointing south. Bend the right knee and adjust your back foot a little further towards the south-east if you wish. You'll notice that the right arm tends to remain roughly in the same position as with the Pull, but the body twists slightly to lead with the outer aspect of the right shoulder – a bit like barging down a door. The left hand, meanwhile, rises a little to about the height of your lower ribs, palm facing slightly forward and down. Although this is a wide stance, the hips and shoulders turn away from the direction of the leading foot and finish up facing south-east.

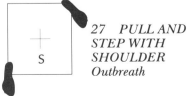

70%

*27 PULL AND STEP WITH SHOULDER*
*Outbreath*

# Crane Spreads Its Wings
## (Photos 28–29)

28   This is another narrow stance and so again it is helpful to adjust what is to become the back, weighted foot first. This time it is the right foot which is going to take the strain, so turn in the foot now. Next, rotate your centre to face the east and draw across the empty left foot to place it down in a narrow toe stance. At the same time raise your right arm, like a great wing, palm looking forward and slightly upwards, as if saluting.

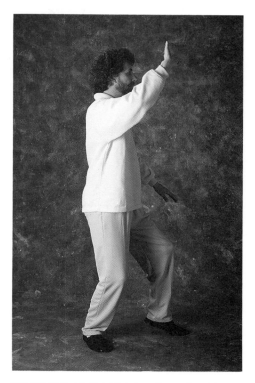

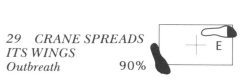

*28   CRANE SPREADS
ITS WINGS
Inbreath*                    *E*

                    90%

29   Lower your right arm, leading with the little finger side of the hand down to about hip height. Simultaneously, commence a vertical clockwise circle with your lower, left hand so that it rises and sweeps around in front of your centre. The whole thing resembles the graceful flapping of gigantic wings, like a great bird drying itself in the sunshine, head, hips and shoulders still all facing east. And that's it! It might seem like an odd place to finish but this movement, perhaps more than any other, has few apparent boundaries between itself and the one that follows.

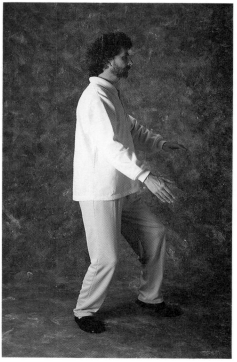

*29   CRANE SPREADS
ITS WINGS
Outbreath*          *E*
                90%

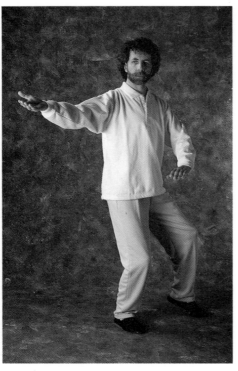

# Brush Left Knee and Push (Photos 30–31)

30   Turn your waist clockwise, almost due south, and simultaneously circle back with your right hand at about chest height. This is a continuation of the wide circling movements of Crane. In a sense you still have wings. The palm should be facing upwards during the intial stages of this movement, rather like holding a custard pie in readiness. That might sound a bit peculiar, but it really is an accurate way of describing the orientation of the palm.

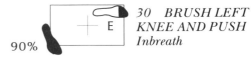

90%

*30   BRUSH LEFT KNEE AND PUSH Inbreath*

31   Now, you are going to take a step forward with the left foot. It is already forward of your right foot anyway, so almost all you need to do is step sideways. The clockwise circle made with your left hand, which you commenced at the end of Crane Spreads Its Wings, continues so that the hand seems to figuratively 'brush' over the left knee toward the north, at a distance of at least six or seven inches between your hand and your thigh. And it is precisely as this 'brushing' of the knee occurs that you take the step with your left heel. Then the right hand comes forward, past your ear, to finally push out eastwards at about chest height.

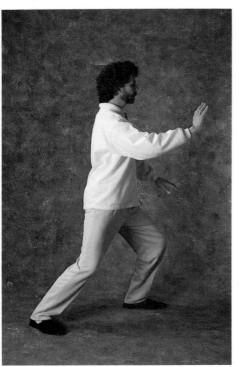

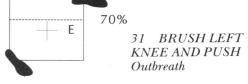

70%

*31   BRUSH LEFT KNEE AND PUSH Outbreath*

# Play Guitar (Left Side) (Photos 32–33)

**32**   Bring all your weight into the left foot and allow the back foot to follow through — leaving the ground and travelling forward a short way. This is the first time one of your feet has actually been off the ground for any length of time — only for a second or so, but it is a good test of how well your sense of balance is progressing. Try turning out the right toes a little as you do this, which is good for the hip joint and ankle.

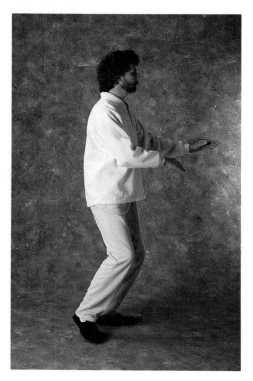

*32   PLAY GUITAR (LEFT SIDE) Inbreath*

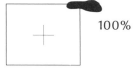

100%

**33**   You are now going to repeat Play Guitar, but on the other side, so that it is now going to be the *left* heel touching the ground and the *left* arm extended furthest from your body rather than the right. Sit back and place the right foot down behind, with a gentle rocking back of the body westwards. Then draw across your left foot into a narrow heel stance, toes still pointing east and make the Play Guitar shape with your arms — left arm leading, and with the palm of your right hand 'looking' at the inside of your left forearm.

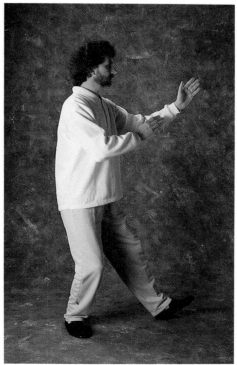

*33   PLAY GUITAR (LEFT SIDE) Outbreath*         90%

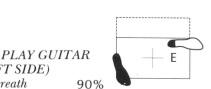

# Brush Left Knee and Push

Next in the sequence we find our first real repetition of movement –
something you have already learned. Here, you need to repeat the
section entitled Brush Knee and Push, so refer back to photos 30 and 31
for this and then simply add it to your sequence, going through it in
exactly the same way as before, only of course you will begin from a left
*heel* stance rather than the left *toe* stance that constituted Crane Spreads
Its Wings. Don't forget to turn the waist southwards as you circle back
with the palm; then step wide, 'brush' the left knee and push out with the
right palm, just as before, head, hips and shoulders all facing east, left
knee over left toes. If in any doubt, refer also to the composite illustration
on pages 112–115 where the entire form is illustrated in miniature.

> **66** *Pay attention to the waist at all times.* **99**
> Tai Chi Classics

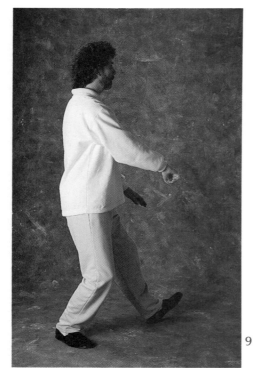

## Step Forward, Parry and Punch (Photos 34–37)

34   We are now embarking on a
forward stepping sequence, heading
eastwards. We do this with a 1–2–3
step; three movements of the feet
which some students find helpful to
count aloud while they are learning.
Begin by shifting your weight back and
turning out the left toes. Lower both
arms to the left side and form a loose
fist with your right hand. Put the left
foot flat and count aloud the number 1
at this point, if it helps.

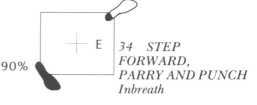

90%   *34   STEP
FORWARD,
PARRY AND PUNCH
Inbreath*

35    With your weight in your left foot, take a step forward with your right and place it down at quite an angle, almost south. Bend the right knee and bring your weight forward, too. At the same time 'throw' the fist over to your right hip, palm side up in readiness for the 'punch'. Count aloud the number 2 if it helps.

*Note:* it is often tempting to speed things up at this stage. Don't. Instead, keep in touch with your breathing and allow the movements to remain smooth and gentle. Try to keep a low centre of gravity as you walk: cat-like.

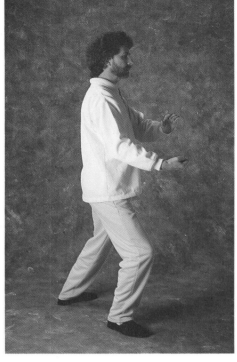

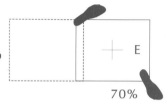

*35    STEP FORWARD, PARRY AND PUNCH*
*Outbreath*

70%

36    Next, raise your left foot and begin to step forward straight to the east. Keep the left hand relaxed and keep the fist in readiness at your right hip. Try drawing in the left toes a little towards the right heel before stepping. Take your time during this; don't get carried away with the idea of the 'punch' you are about to deliver. Remember the tai chi form is always done in a spirit of calm and relaxation.

*Note:* the left hand is not idle during all of this. Keep the palm open and soft, but allow it to follow your right fist a little, around towards the centre.

*36    STEP FORWARD, PARRY AND PUNCH*
*Inbreath*

100%

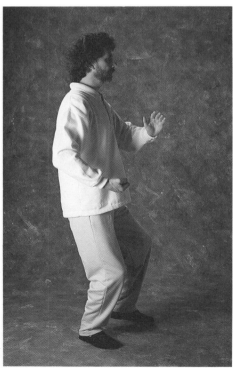

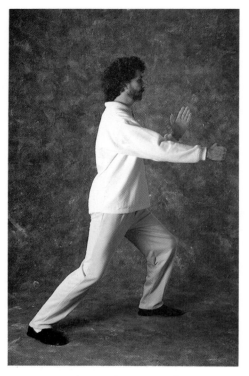

37   Now place the left heel down and bend the left knee, the foot facing directly east. Count aloud the number 3 if you like. At the same time, parry with your left arm or, in other words, raise the forearm to a near vertical position in front of your body, allowing it to swing out slightly left of centre, as if deflecting an oncoming force. Then, project the fist slowly forward towards the east, finishing at about the height of the solar plexus – no higher. This is your 'punch', but do it very slowly, for the duration of one whole outbreath.

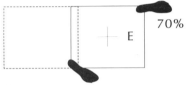

*37   STEP FORWARD,
PARRY AND PUNCH
Outbreath*

## Release Arm and Push (Photos 38–40)

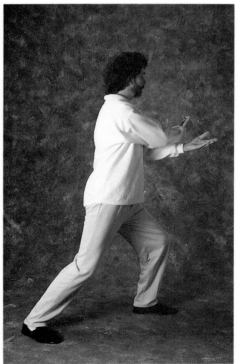

38   This next movement is a little intricate but highly beneficial for the joints of the wrists and elbows. With a slight counter-clockwise turning of the waist, slide the fingers of your left hand underneath your right forearm. Keep a little space between your hand and forearm – no contact – and keep those shoulders open and relaxed!

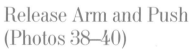

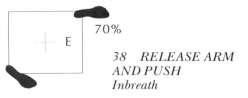

*38   RELEASE ARM
AND PUSH
Inbreath*

39   Open the fist and turn palms up.
Then, shifting your weight back into
the right foot, draw your right arm
back also, across on top of your left
forearm. The waist turns a little
clockwise as you do this. Finally, rotate
the palms inwards. Keep both feet flat
on the ground and make sure your
spine remains vertical. Do not lean
back! Relax the wrists as you rotate the
hands, always making sure the hands
or the forearms do not touch each
other. Take your time, rotating very
slowly, very smoothly.

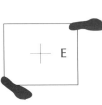

*39   RELEASE ARM*
*AND PUSH*           70%
*Inbreath finishes*

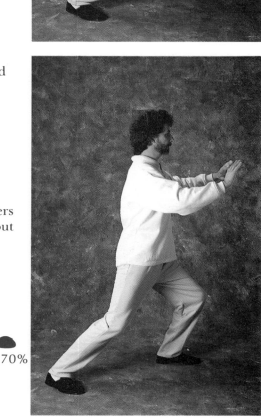

40   Rotate the palms slowly to face
outwards. Bring your weight forward
once again by bending the left knee
and push forward with both hands.
This double-handed push is very
similar to the one you did earlier on
(see page 27), but this time you have
your *left* leg forward, of course, and
you are facing the east. Again, your
push should be no higher than the
level of your chest. Keep the shoulders
relaxed and the spine straight, without
leaning forward.

*40   RELEASE ARM*
*AND PUSH*
*Outbreath*

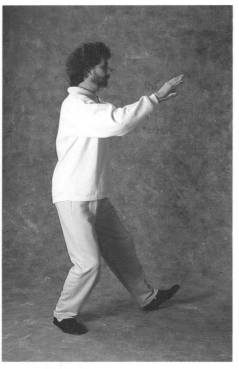

# Turn and Close Part One (Photos 41–45)

41    Sit back once again onto the rear foot, but this time a fraction further so that you can raise your left toes a little. Everything remains facing east at this stage – the palms still turned out, though slightly more relaxed than when they were pushing. This is a Yin, retreating movement, so let your hands reflect that quality by softening slightly and relaxing at the wrists. The aspect of the hands is, I think, a little like somebody warming their hands at the fireside.

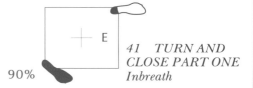

90%

*41    TURN AND CLOSE PART ONE Inbreath*

42    Now, pivot on your left heel to get the toes facing south. Let your centre turn towards the south also. Once you are there, you should be starting to breathe out. Up until now the hands have remained more or less in the push position but now they are starting to separate and move outwards from each other, initially in a wide arc but in a moment this is going to become a full circle.

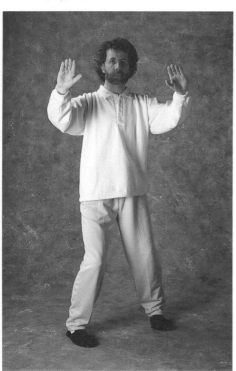

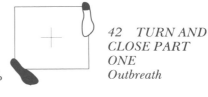

90%

*42    TURN AND CLOSE PART ONE Outbreath*

43    Bring all your weight into the left
leg as the hands continue to circle
outwards and downwards to your
sides. The hands are actually in the
process of making a large circle in
front of you, the right hand moving
out and down to the west, clockwise,
and the left hand moving out and
down to the east, counter-clockwise.
You should be getting to the end of
your outbreath now.

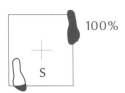

*43    TURN AND
CLOSE PART
ONE
Outbreath finishes*

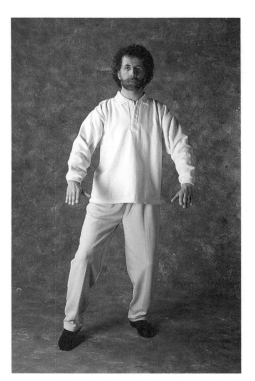

44    Once you feel you are properly
balanced in your left foot, draw back
the right foot to place it alongside, with
the toes also facing south. The hands
have reached their lowest point, at
your sides, but with the next inbreath
they start to rise again up through
your centre, palms in, until they cross,
left wrist resting upon the right, at
about the height of your chin. The
weight becomes evenly distributed
again here at the close of Part One,
and you should be finding a state of
equilibrium between the two feet.

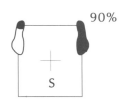

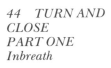

*44    TURN AND
CLOSE
PART ONE
Inbreath*

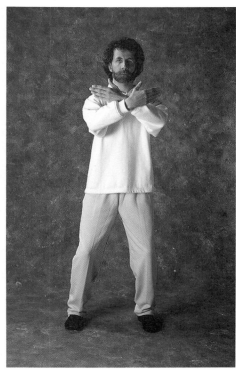

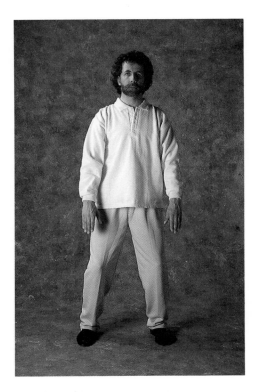

45    All that remains to conclude Part One is to lower your arms gently down through your centre to rest at your sides, separating naturally as they fall. Breathe out, sink down, relax the knees and allow the shoulders and fingers to relax also. If this is as far as you wish to go – i.e. just Part One – then take a few deep breaths to finish, experiencing how the body feels for a moment before moving away.

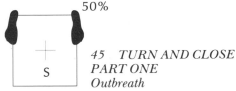

*45    TURN AND CLOSE*
*PART ONE*
*Outbreath*

*Note:* if and when you proceed to Part Two, you will need to make a slight alteration to the ending of this movement. This, however, does not concern you at this stage and it will be described at the start of the next chapter.

> **❝** *Reproach no man with imperfections, taught our master; do you not see that he is taking the greatest trouble to make progress – be it ever so little.* **❞**
> Selvarajan Yesudian

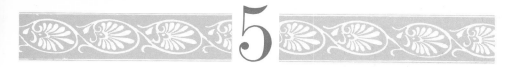

# 5

# THE FORM – PART TWO

> 66 *Hold fast to it and you can keep it; let go and it will stray. For its comings and goings it has no time nor tide; none knows where it will bide.* 99
>
> Confucius

## Step-by-step instructions

### Carry Tiger to Mountain (Photos 46–47)

46  From your crossed hands position at the end of Part One, sink onto the left leg. Then, rather than lowering your arms down to your sides to finish, as you did before, drop them down to your left side, the back of your left hand brushing, at a distance, the back of your right as you separate the hands at waist height. Raise the right heel and pivot a little on the toes, allowing the waist to commence its turn clockwise, in readiness for a big step around to the north-west. Then slowly raise the left hand, palm up, to shoulder height.

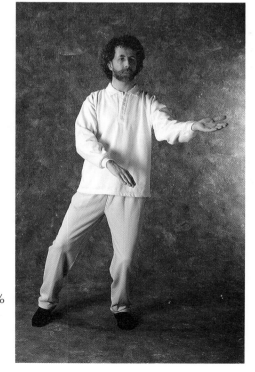

 90%

*46  CARRY TIGER TO MOUNTAIN*
*Inbreath*

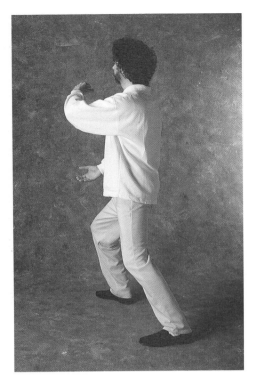

47 Step around with your right foot to place it down, heel first, towards the north-west. At the same time, 'brush' the right knee with your right palm and bring the left hand around above it. Bring your weight into the right leg by bending the knee and finally turn your right palm up, as if supporting a large ball, the left hand on top, head, hips and shoulders all facing north-west.

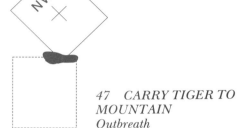

70%

NW

47   CARRY TIGER TO
MOUNTAIN
*Outbreath*

## Diagonal Rollback, Diagonal Press, Diagonal Separate Hands and Push, Diagonal Single Whip

If you think of the tai chi form as a piece of music, then what comes next could be termed 'The Chorus', a sequence of movements that you learned in Part One and which you will find repeated three more times here in Part Two. The Chorus normally consists of Grasp Bird's Tail through to Single Whip – though just at this particular place, we will miss out Grasp Bird's Tail, beginning the whole thing with Rollback.

You can slip into Rollback quite easily from the previous position by simply sitting back onto your rear leg, raising the right arm and 'cupping' the elbow with your left hand – everything the same as the Rollback in Part One, only facing north-west instead of west. After that, continue with Press, Separate Hands and Push, and the Single Whip. For all these, refer to photos 13 to 23, or to the composite illustration on pages 112–115.

At the conclusion of your Diagonal Single Whip you will, of course, be facing south-east instead of east. The foot diagram given here indicates where you should be. Head, hips and shoulders are facing south-east, left knee over left toes.

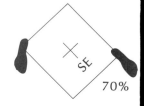

SE

70%

# Fist Under Elbow
# (Photos 48–50)

**48**   You are now going to get yourself back onto the east/west axis with some neat footwork. In all, there are just three movements of the feet and it might help you to count them out loud, just as I suggested earlier with Step Forward, Parry and Punch.

Following the Diagonal Single Whip, sit back onto your right leg and open up the hands in a relaxed fashion. Pivot on your empty left heel and point your left toes to the east. Let the foot go flat on the ground and count the number 1 out loud.

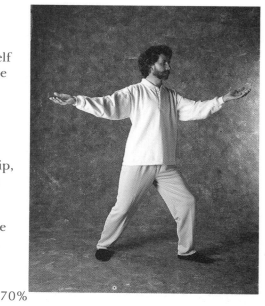

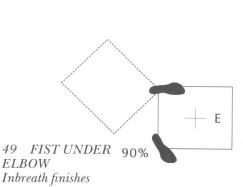

70%

*48   FIST UNDER ELBOW*
*Inbreath*

**49**   Next, with all your weight now in the left foot, slowly draw up your right foot alongside it, with the toes pointing outwards. Count aloud the number 2 as your weight flows into the right side. At the same time your arms drop and then circle round to your left side, covering your centre. Your inbreath is coming to a conclusion now.

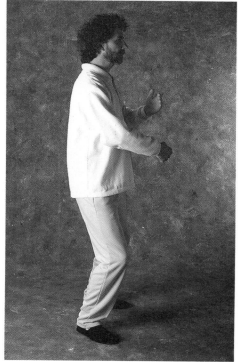

E

*49   FIST UNDER ELBOW*  90%
*Inbreath finishes*

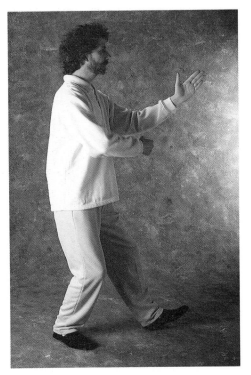

50   Bring all your weight into your right foot and slide forward and inwards with your left foot to form a narrow heel stance to the east, counting aloud the number 3. Simultaneously, project your left arm forward, almost 'threading' it through the palm of your right hand. Finally, make the right hand into a loose fist which settles just beneath and slightly to the inside of your left elbow, abdomen height. By this time, your head, hips and shoulders should all be facing east. Let your eyes settle upon an imaginary distant horizon, looking over the tips of your left fingers and make sure your right wrist is relaxed.

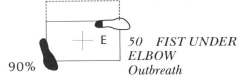

90%

50   *FIST UNDER ELBOW*
*Outbreath*

## Repulse Monkey (Right Side) (Photos 51–53)

51   With your weight still in the back leg, let go of your fist and turn up the left palm. There is a little story attached to this sequence which assists in memorising the actions. Imagine you are face to face with a monkey (the monkey is in fact a much-respected deity in parts of the Orient and is a creature credited with much wisdom as well as playfulness). You are going to offer him some food in the palm of your left hand. This is the 'purpose' of turning the left palm up. At the same time circle your right palm back, rather like you did at the beginning stages of Brush Knee and Push.

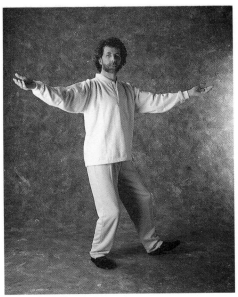

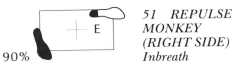

90%

51   *REPULSE MONKEY (RIGHT SIDE)*
*Inbreath*

52   Raise your left foot and draw it back. You are actually in the process of stepping backwards here as the monkey advances to take the food. The right palm, in the meantime, has rotated and is beginning to face forward. As the foot continues to go back, allow the left hand to drop, very slowly towards your left hip, keeping the palm open and relaxed and the elbow out, away from your ribs.

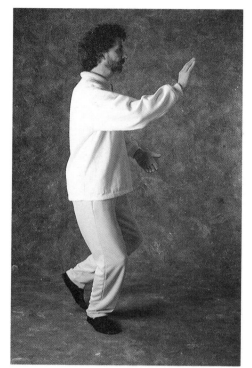

*52   REPULSE MONKEY*
*(RIGHT SIDE)*
*Inbreath finishes*        100%

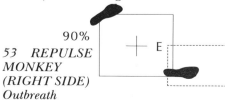

53   Place the left foot down behind you, making contact with the toes first. Withdraw your left hand entirely now, down to the level of your waist, just as the monkey is coming to grab the food. The right palm meanwhile has just passed your ear and has advanced forward to push the monkey's nose away. The left leg stepping back and the right palm pushing forward all take place at the same time, and are, therefore, completely co-ordinated.

Finally, adjust your right foot by pivoting on your right heel so that the toes face east. Though most of your weight is in the back leg, both feet are actually flat on the ground.

90%

*53   REPULSE*
*MONKEY*
*(RIGHT SIDE)*
*Outbreath*

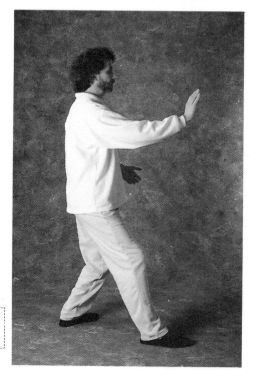

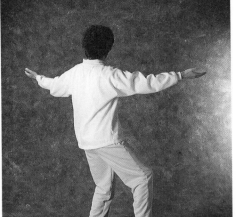

## Repulse Monkey (Left Side) (Photos 54–55)

**54**   You are now going to repeat the whole Repulse Monkey routine once again, but this time starting with the right foot and the right palm forward, so that you will eventually step back onto your right foot. Begin by 'offering the food' by turning your right palm up. The left palm meanwhile starts its circle back, palm up, behind your left shoulder.

100%

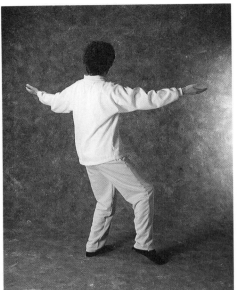

*54   REPULSE MONKEY (LEFT SIDE)*
*Inbreath*

**55**   Just like before, you step back, toes first, this time with the right foot and at the same time withdraw your right palm down to the level of your waist. The left palm then circles forward to push the monkey's nose away again, just as he is about to seize the food. Finally, adjust the front foot by pivoting on the heel. The left toes, head, hips and shoulders are all facing east.

*55   REPULSE MONKEY (LEFT SIDE)*
*Outbreath*

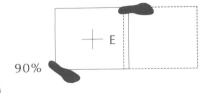

90%

## Repulse Monkey (Right Side)

Here, you simply repeat the first Repulse Monkey routine, so refer to photos 51–53. The only difference is that this time both your feet start off from a position flat on the ground, whereas photo 51 shows the toes of the left foot raised. Go through the whole routine again stepping back with the left foot; withdrawing the left hand; pushing the monkey's nose with your right palm and straightening the right foot by pivoting on the heel.

# Diagonal Flying
# (Photos 56–57)

**56** With most of your weight in the left foot, turn the waist anti-clockwise and allow your right heel to follow – this relieves any strain that might result in the right knee from turning the body away from it. Form a ball, left hand on top, palm down; right hand supporting underneath, palm up. Sink well down into the left foot and prepare to raise the right.

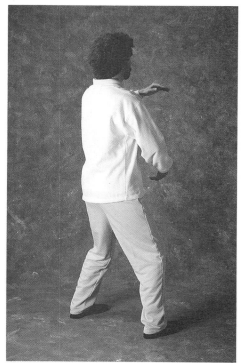

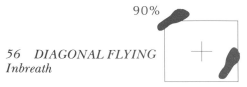

*56  DIAGONAL FLYING*
*Inbreath*

**57** Lift your right foot from the ground, turn the waist clockwise and direct your right hip around – way around, so that you can put your right heel down with the toes pointing as near to the south-west as possible. This is another one of those big steps, like Carry Tiger to Mountain, and it is vital, therefore, as soon as the weight starts to shift into the right foot, that you adjust the rear, left, foot to a comfortable angle by pivoting on the heel. The arms, meanwhile, separate out, with the right arm 'flying' around to the south-west in a slanting-upwards aspect and the left hand sinking down to the left hip, palm down and slightly backward facing.

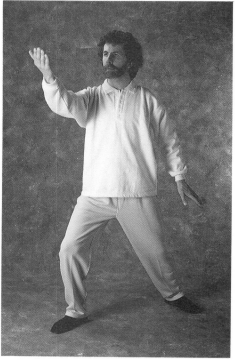

*57  DIAGONAL*
*FLYING*
*Outbreath*

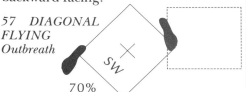

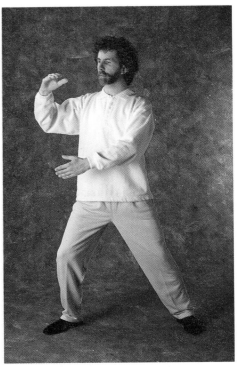

# Cloudy Hands (Introduction) (Photos 58–59)

58   We are now embarking on a really classic set of movements – Cloudy Hands (sometimes also called 'Wave Hands Like Clouds'). The first thing to do is to re-align yourself with the east/west axis and to do this you simply draw up the rear (left) foot. It is important that it is placed down a good distance from your right, however; something in the order of between one and a half to double shoulder width. At the same time, keep your weight flowing into the right leg and sweep your left hand round and beneath your right hand.

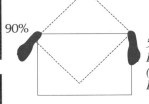

90%

*58   CLOUDY HANDS (INTRODUCTION) Inbreath*

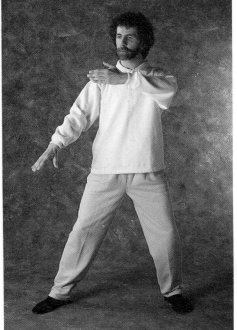

59   Start to shift your weight into the left leg and change the hands over; that is, lower the right hand down and slightly outwards to hip level while simultaneously raising the left hand to about shoulder level. The left hand rises inside the right – or in other words, closer to your body than the right. The actions of the hands are very soft – like describing the shapes of billowing clouds in the air.

70%

S

*59   CLOUDY HANDS (INTRODUCTION) Outbreath*

# Cloudy Hands (Left)
# (Photos 60–62)

60  With most of your weight now in
the left leg, pivot on your right heel so
that the toes point south. The feet are
therefore parallel. At the same time,
draw your right palm around to face
inwards to your centre, at about
abdomen height. Your left palm
should also be facing in by this stage, at
about the height of your throat, in a
line above your right hand. You can be
commencing your inbreath at this
point.

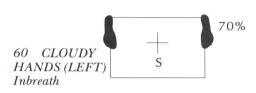

70%

*60  CLOUDY
HANDS (LEFT)*
*Inbreath*

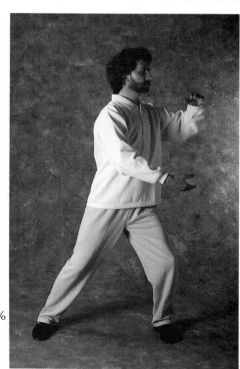

61  Next, turn the waist anti-
clockwise, bringing the arms around
with your centre, and form a ball with
the hands. Your weight will naturally
want to concentrate in the left foot as
you do this. Keep the knees apart, as if
sitting on a horse, but make sure they
remain flexible. Also, make sure that
your hips (and therefore the arms, too)
only turn as far as you naturally feel
they want to go. If you sense the
muscles in your waist and back
knotting up or your knees caving in
towards each other, then you have
gone too far.

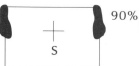

90%

*61  CLOUDY
HANDS (LEFT)*
*Inbreath finishes*

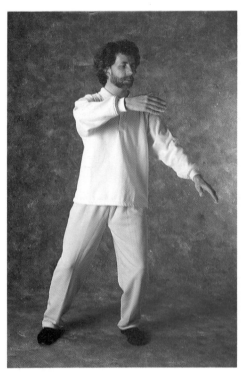

62   Now empty the right foot entirely and bring it inwards towards the left, closing in to about shoulder width. At the same time change the hands over, by bringing the right hand up to shoulder height and letting the left hand fall to about hip height. As with the previous change of hands (photo 59) it is the lower hand which rises inside the upper hand, or in other words the right hand rises closer to your side than the left. Think of the top hand pushing out a little to the east to make room for it.

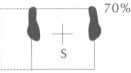

62   CLOUDY
HANDS (LEFT)
*Outbreath*

## Cloudy Hands (Right) (Photos 63–65)

63   You next repeat the sequence on the other side. So rotate your waist back to face south and position your hands as before, though this time with the right hand facing in at throat level, the left hand beneath it, facing in at abdomen level. Again, try to direct the movements of the arms via the waist and make sure those knees remain apart! The free turning of the waist is the key to these movements and is probably why Cloudy Hands is considered to be so beneficial in terms of aiding the digestive organs.

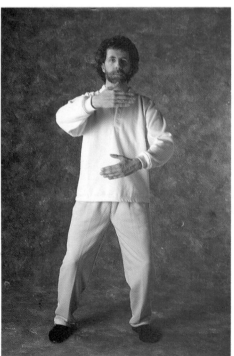

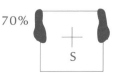

63   CLOUDY
HANDS (RIGHT)
*Inbreath*

64 Keep turning the waist clockwise as far as you can comfortably go and form a ball with the hands again, this time with the right hand on top, left hand underneath. Most of your weight will want to settle in the right leg as you go. Keep your waist and diaphragm – the large muscle under the ribs that assists in breathing – as relaxed as possible during these movements. If necessary, take time off and gently press your finger tips under and around the lower rib cage and abdomen to help loosen things. Gently please! Don't prod, just press lightly. Then return to the movement and see if it feels any different.

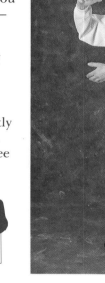

90%

64 CLOUDY HANDS
(RIGHT)
Inbreath finishes

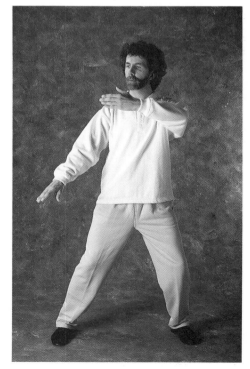

65 Empty the left foot entirely and step with it away from your right foot – i.e. eastwards – settling at about one and a half to double shoulder width distance, the toes still continuing to point south. At the same time change hands again, this time by bringing the left hand up to shoulder height and letting the right hand fall to about hip height. And again, if it helps, think of the top hand pushing out a little to the west to make room for the lower one to rise in its place.

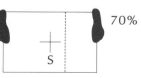

65 CLOUDY
HANDS
(RIGHT)
Outbreath

70%

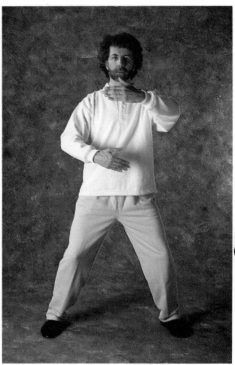

# Cloudy Hands (Left Into Whip) (Photos 66–68)

66   Although Cloudy Hands Left has been illustrated before (60–62) we are going to look at it again here because at the end of it there is an important variation with which we gain access to the next movement. So turn your centre to face south and position the hands as before – left hand on top, throat height, right hand underneath, abdomen height.

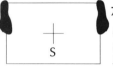

70%

*66   CLOUDY HANDS (LEFT INTO WHIP)*
*Inbreath*

67   Keep turning the waist anti-clockwise, again as far as you can comfortably go. Form a ball with the hands, left hand on top. Most of your weight will want to settle in the left leg, as before. Through all these movements, just let the hands 'float'. Imagine your forearms and hands have become feather-like, gently undulating through the air or, cloud-like, soft, graceful and rounded. Imagine your internal energy is holding the arms up, rather than muscle power.

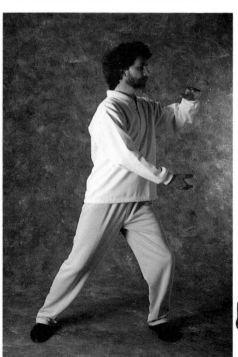

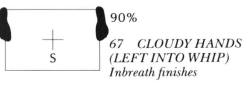

90%

*67   CLOUDY HANDS (LEFT INTO WHIP)*
*Inbreath finishes*

68   Now to conclude the sequence. At this point you are, of course, in the position where you are ready to step and change once again. But this time as you change you do not step in with your right foot but forwards, just half a pace. Then, as you change, and as you draw up that right hand, you do so with it shaped into a Crane's Beak – the same hook shape that you used in the Single Whip earlier. You have, in fact, broken half-way into what is to become a Single Whip; so the left palm will want to turn up as well in readiness for the completion of the movement to the east, which is precisely what happens next.

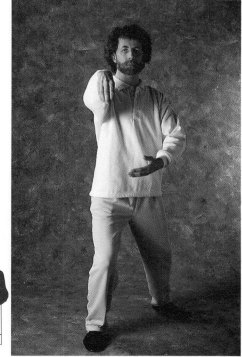

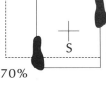

*68   CLOUDY HANDS*
*(LEFT INTO WHIP)*
*Outbreath*          70%

# Isolated Single Whip
# (Photos 69–70)

69   From the previous position, which left you in the process of exiting from Cloudy Hands, you continue by emptying the rear foot and raising it from the ground. Breathe in and start to be aware of the step you are going to take towards the east. Look at your left palm.

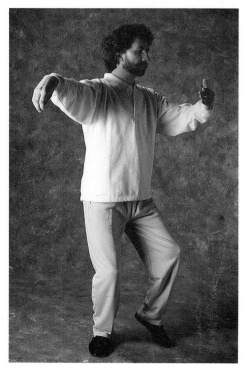

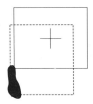

*69   ISOLATED*
*SINGLE WHIP*          100%
*Inbreath*

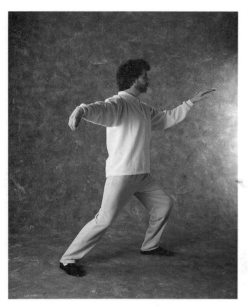

70   Finish off this isolated Single Whip ('isolated' because it occurs outside the context of 'The Chorus') by placing the left heel down to the east and bringing up the left hand to point the fingers east. Make sure you have stepped into a proper 70/30 stance. Bend the left knee and adjust the right heel to a comfortable position, head, hips and shoulders all facing east, left knee over left toes. Keep that left elbow relaxed and your wrist, too.

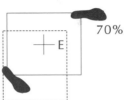

*70   ISOLATED SINGLE WHIP*
*Outbreath*

## Snake Creeps Down (Photos 71–72)

71   This movement – a classical piece much beloved by painters and sculptors – is sometimes called a Squatting Single Whip because your Crane's Beak, left over from the Single Whip, remains intact throughout. To begin, you will need to create a bit more length between your feet. So slide or shuffle (depending on the kind of surface you're on) back a little with your right foot and turn on your heel to get your right toes pointing back towards the south-west. Then pivot on your left heel and get your left toes pointing in, roughly to the south-east. As your inbreath finishes start to sink back and downwards, squatting onto your left foot. Keep that right arm extended.

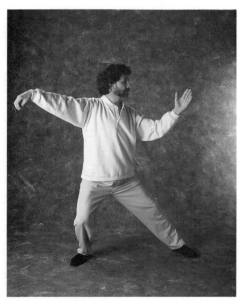

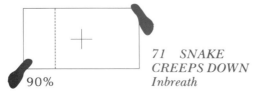

*71   SNAKE CREEPS DOWN*
*Inbreath*

72   Breathe out and continue sinking back. The left hand meanwhile is drawn in towards your chest, the fingers close together. Keep it going, on down through your centre, dipping in a great arc to the floor, almost scraping the ground at its lowest point and then on forward towards your left foot – by now with the palm facing south. Then, as it brushes past your left foot, not touching it, it is as though it pushes the left foot straight – the foot turning back on its heel to point the toes due east once again.

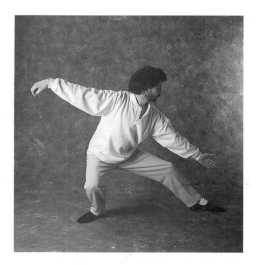

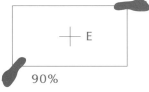

*72   SNAKE CREEPS DOWN Outbreath*

## Golden Pheasant (Right Side) (Photos 73–74)

73   Now here is a test for your balance. Up until now you have always had the tip of a toe or a heel on the ground when your weight has been wholly in one leg but here you actually raise the insubstantial leg right off the ground. The whole movement emulates the proud actions of a cock bird raising one leg. Firstly, however, you need to extricate yourself from Snake Creeps Down and it is surprising how many people have problems with this. Follow these simple steps and you will be able to perform the movement smoothly.

Firstly, bring your right foot back to its comfortable, south-east facing position. Turn out the left foot by pivoting on your left heel, then bring the weight slowly forward and bend your left knee. From here it is easy to come up into the one-legged posture of Golden Pheasant.

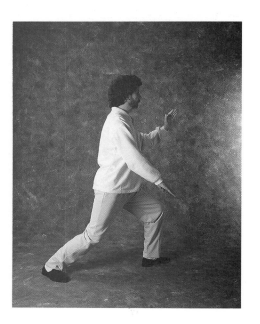

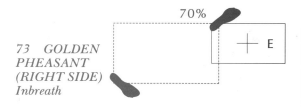

*73   GOLDEN PHEASANT (RIGHT SIDE) Inbreath*

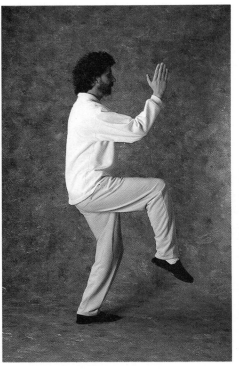

74   So, now straighten the body and draw up the right knee and right hand, fingers pointing up. Think of a cock bird, standing on one leg. This is very much a contrast to the downward, mysterious Snake we encountered just a moment ago. Here everything is very 'up front' and showy. If at first you have trouble balancing, don't worry. Just keep your toe in contact with the ground. As long as you at least try to bring your focus of balance into the substantial leg, and as long as you can raise your right heel from the ground, you will have made a good start. Gradually, your balance will improve.

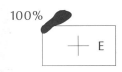

*74   GOLDEN PHEASANT (RIGHT SIDE)*
*Inbreath finishes*

## Golden Pheasant (Left Side) (Photos 75–76)

75   You are now about to reverse the previous posture. Start by placing your right foot down with the toes pointing south-east and then transfer all your weight into it. At the same time allow the right arm to fall naturally to your side. Do this very slowly, under control. If you feel you have to lunge or stumble down, then you are not cultivating the right degree of balance. Keep it smooth!

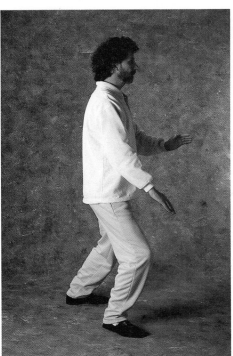

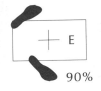

*75   GOLDEN PHEASANT (LEFT SIDE)*
*Outbreath*

76   Slowly raising the left knee and left arm, you next perform the same actions, emulating the cock bird, but this time on the other side. Try a very subtle scuffing of the ground with your toes as they come up – just like the cock bird, if you care to watch him sometime. Try to really evoke the spirit of the creature. Be part of it.

   I sometimes ask my students to think of a Swiss penknife when they practise this movement. This is because the leg and arm should be aligned in one plane, i.e. the hand, elbow, knee, shin and foot all arranged with their leading edges facing due east. It's worthwhile getting somebody to check this for you occasionally, to make sure the limbs are not deviating.

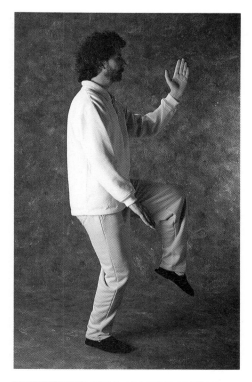

*76   GOLDEN
PHEASANT
(LEFT SIDE)
Inbreath*

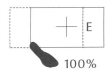

E

100%

## Pat The Horse (Right) (Photo 77)

77   Place your left foot down slightly behind you, toes first, and allow your centre to rotate naturally towards the leading foot, i.e. south-east. At the same time imagine you have a horse or – more accurately, I always think – a pony there at your side. Place your right hand on its neck and hold an apple for him to eat in your left palm. This will get you more or less into the correct position – though in practice, you should eventually be aiming to make the movement more flowing, with the left palm sliding down along the right forearm somewhat as you sweep up and across with the right hand.

90%

*77   PAT THE HORSE
(RIGHT)
Outbreath*

SE

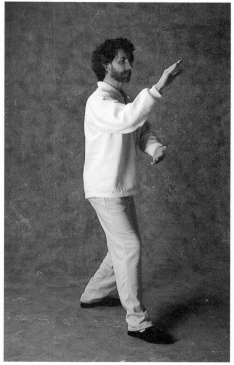

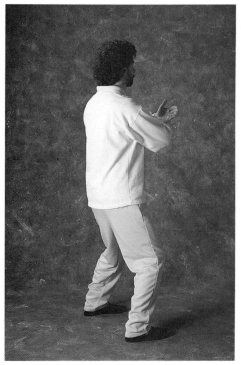

## Kick With Right Toes (Photos 78–79)

78 Further one-legged action here, with the first of two toe kicks. First, however, you need to gather your arms into a cross shape which will then separate out, forwards and backwards, just before you kick. To do this, turn on your right heel to go very slightly pigeon-toed. Your centre now faces north-east. Next, lower the right hand and place the right wrist underneath your left at about abdomen height. Then roll the wrists up, so that the palms face outwards (north-east). Simultaneously, draw up the right knee in readiness for your kick.

90%

*78 KICK WITH RIGHT TOES*
*Inbreath*

79 Separate the hands – the right hand going forwards, south-east, and the left hand going back behind, travelling in a great arc, finishing at shoulder height. Then straighten the rest of your leg and make a kicking motion with your right toes, out towards the south-east in a line with your right arm. The height of this kick is not important. But do draw up the knee before you kick and only bring it up as high as is realistic and comfortable for you. If you bring it up too high, you will tend to fall back as you complete the kick.

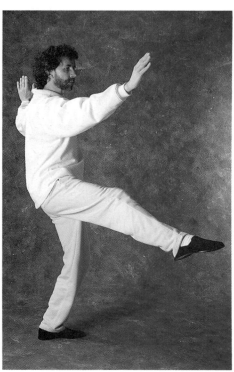

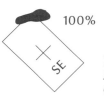

100%

*79 KICK WITH RIGHT TOES*
*Outbreath*

# Pat The Horse (Left) (Photos 80–81)

80    You are now going to pat the pony again, only this time with your left hand. But first, directly following the kick and with the knee still up, you need to take an inbreath and let the shin drop into a relaxed position. Your palms tend to face in towards each other at this stage, in preparation for the next move. This pattern of breathing in directly after a kick and prior to the next Yang movement is typical of the tai chi form.

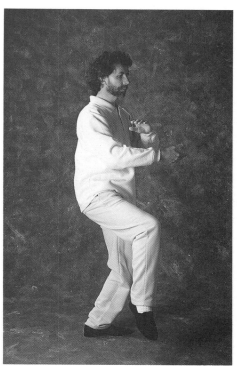

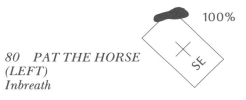

100%

*80    PAT THE HORSE (LEFT)*
*Inbreath*

81    Place the right heel down, again facing south-east and a little ahead of your left foot. The pony has moved around to your left side this time so, as you put the foot down, it is your left hand which you place on the pony's neck while the right hand, palm up, is the one that holds the apple. Again, once you have learned the basic 'nuts and bolts' of this manoeuvre, try to get the hands to flow more gracefully with the right palm loosely sliding – at a distance – along the edge of the left forearm as it comes back and down to your centre, both hands moving in graceful, continuous arcs, the fingers relaxed.

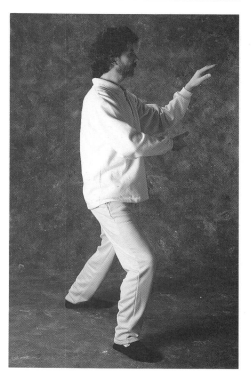

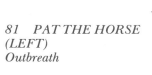

*81    PAT THE HORSE (LEFT)*
*Outbreath*

90%

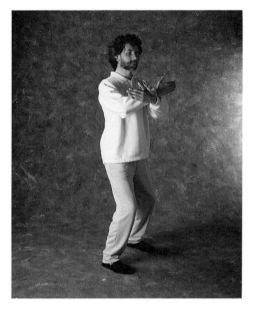

# Kick With Left Toes (Photos 82–83)

**82**   Step up with your left foot alongside your right and start thinking in terms of a toe kick, rather like the one you did before but this time to the north-east. First, however, you need to gather up your arms into another one of those crossed formations which will then separate out again, one hand forwards, one hand backwards, just prior to the kick. To do this, turn on your left heel, going very slightly pigeon-toed; then lower the left hand and place the left wrist underneath your right at about abdomen height. Then roll the wrists up, so that the palms face outwards (south-east) and simultaneously, draw up the left knee in readiness for your kick.

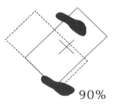

90%

*82   KICK WITH LEFT TOES*
*Inbreath*

**83**   Separate the hands, with the left hand going forwards, north-east, and the right hand travelling back behind. Then draw up the rest of your leg and make a very slow, gentle and controlled kicking motion with your left toes, out towards the north-east.

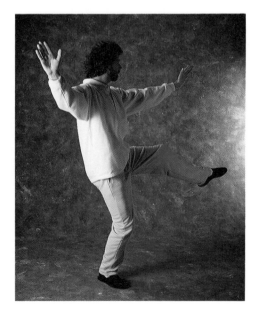

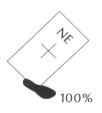

100%

*83   KICK WITH LEFT TOES*
*Outbreath*

# Turn and Kick With The Sole (Photos 84–85)

**84**   This is a movement that can seem quite tricky when you first encounter it but it is – like most tai chi movements – 99% technique. You are going to turn around to the west on the heel of your right foot whilst keeping the left foot entirely off the ground. That successfully completed, you finish by kicking out to the west with the left foot. Here's how.

After the previous position, do not put the left foot down at all. Instead, just lower the shin into a vertical position. Drop the arms also, the left arm vertical through the middle of the body, the right just outside your right thigh. Then using the momentum of your left leg and right arm, turn anti-clockwise on your right heel so that the right toes face north-west. Your hips and shoulders go round a bit further, to face due west.

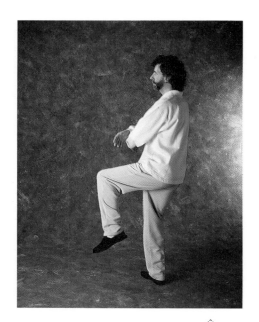

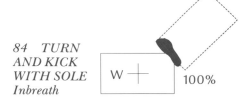

*84   TURN AND KICK WITH SOLE Inbreath*   W   100%

**85**   Now gather up the hands in that by now familiar cross shape. Sources differ as to which wrist crosses which at this stage but I prefer to allow the right wrist to cross naturally over the left during the course of the turn. Then raise the arms so that the palms turn out northwards. Separate the hands again – left hand westward, right hand back behind you – and then kick, as slowly as you can, with the sole of the left foot out to the west. Don't rush into this. Make sure you have turned successfully and have settled down in your right leg first.

*85   TURN AND KICK WITH SOLE Outbreath*

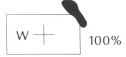

W   100%

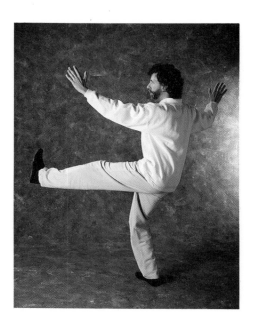

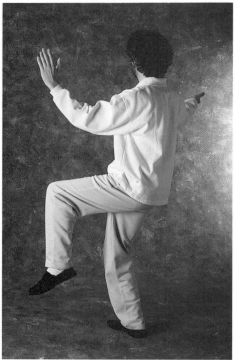

# Brush Left Knee and Push (Photos 86–87)

86 We have encountered this movement before, in Part One. However, it is illustrated again here since the lead-in to it is slightly different – for one thing, the left foot is above the ground. After the kick, drop the shin, keeping the thigh horizontal. Take an inbreath, then bring back the left arm above your knee – the appearance here being, for a moment, not unlike another Golden Pheasant. The right hand, however, is behind you, not at your side; and it turns, palm up, in readiness to push forward to the west.

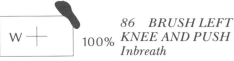

100%

*86 BRUSH LEFT KNEE AND PUSH Inbreath*

87 Commence your exhalation and place the heel down, under control, ahead of your right foot and shoulder width from it. Bend the left knee to bring the weight forward as you push out with the right palm at about chest height to the west. At the same time the left hand will brush the left knee – see photo 31 for a view of how this looks from the other side.

*Note:* it is important not to stumble or fall into this movement. Always take that inbreath and prepare (Yin) before placing the left foot down slowly and deliberately completing the movement (Yang).

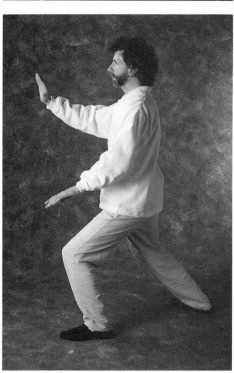

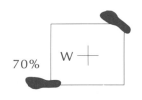

70%

*87 BRUSH LEFT KNEE AND PUSH Outbreath*

# Brush Right Knee and Push (Photos 88–89)

88 Sit back, turn out the left toes by pivoting on the heel. Relax the right hand by turning the palm down somewhat and turn the left palm upwards, so that the hands form a kind of diagonal ball. Breathe in and start to turn your centre anti-clockwise. Let the left hand circle back, still with the palm up. This is, as you have probably guessed, going to be a mirror image of the previous movement. So prepare to step forward with the right foot.

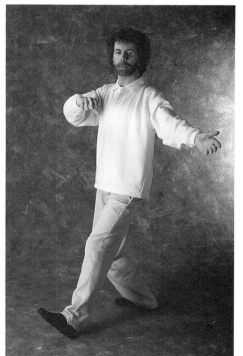

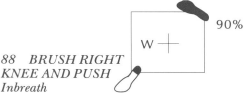

*88  BRUSH RIGHT KNEE AND PUSH*
*Inbreath*

89 Step straight ahead with the right heel to the west and brush the right knee with the right palm, i.e. travelling in a northerly direction. Bring your left hand forward past your ear and then push out with the palm to the west, chest height, as you bend the right knee and bring your weight forward, head, hips and shoulders all facing west, right knee over right toes.

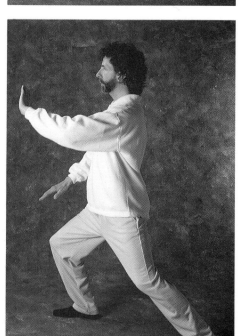

*89  BRUSH RIGHT KNEE AND PUSH*
*Outbreath*

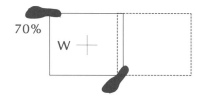

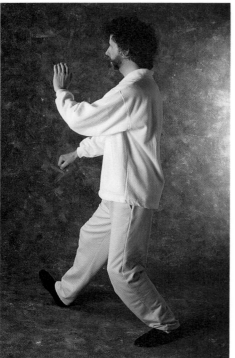

# Brush Left Knee and Punch Low (Photos 90–91)

90    For the next movement, you are going to take another step forward, employing the same style of footwork – that is, turning out what is to become the back foot before stepping forward and so on. This is very similar to Brush Left Knee and Push, except that you do not push out with the right hand at the end but instead very slowly punch low with your right fist.

Begin, then, by sitting back once again and turning out the right toes by pivoting on the heel. Make a loose fist with your right hand and circle it out to your right side.

*90    BRUSH KNEE AND PUNCH LOW*
*Inbreath*

W +

90%

91    Place your left foot forward, pointing west – if you like, drawing in the left toes towards the right foot a little first. At the same time, brush your left knee with your left palm and bring your weight forward by bending your left knee. Allow your body weight to sink down at this point, really low. As this occurs, spiral your right fist down diagonally to about knee height in a slow punching action which finishes with the thumb side of your fist uppermost.

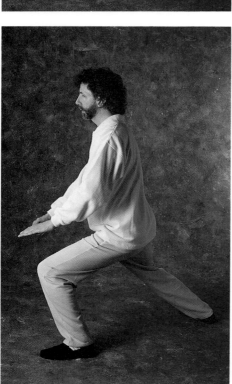

*91    BRUSH LEFT KNEE AND PUNCH LOW*
*Outbreath*

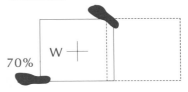

70%    W +

# Grasp Bird's Tail
## (Photos 92–93)

92    We are now about to step into our
third Chorus, this time beginning with
Grasp Bird's Tail. The lead-in to it is
slightly different from what we have
met with before. We do start, however,
with that by now familiar preparation
of sitting back momentarily and
turning out what is to become the back
foot – i.e. pivoting on the left heel to
get the toes out – and then bringing all
of the weight into it. Allow the waist to
follow, turning slightly anti-clockwise,
and then pick up a ball, swooping
under with the right hand to support
the ball from beneath.

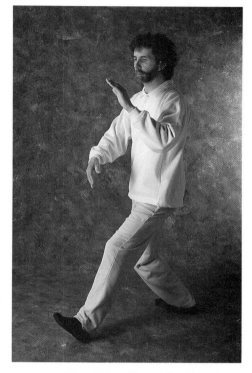

90%

*92    GRASP*
*BIRD'S TAIL*
*Inbreath*

93    Now step forward with the right
heel and bend the knee. At the same
time, raise the right hand up to the
level of your chest, the arm slanting
upwards slightly and position your left
hand so that the fingers are pointing
towards the right palm, adjusting the
left foot to a comfortable position by
pivoting on the heel afterwards. This
turning in of the back foot by pivoting
on the heel is something you should
always aim for when you complete a
forward step into a wide stance, even if
only a tiny bit. The ease or otherwise
with which you can do this often
depends on how well you have set up
the step in the first place – i.e. how far
you originally turned out the back toes
before stepping.

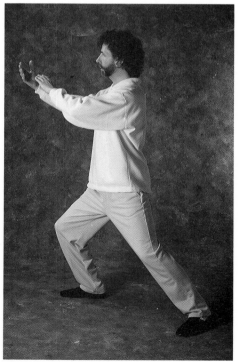

70%

*93    GRASP BIRD'S*
*TAIL*
*Outbreath*

## Rollback, Press, Separate Hands and Push, Single Whip

Continuing with your Chorus, repeat once again all the above movements. Refer to photos 13–23 or to the composite drawing on pages 112–115 if in any doubt. The Single Whip, however, will ultimately take you into a wide 70/30 stance, facing east, from where we will take up our instructions once again.

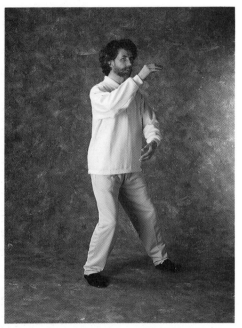

## Four Corners (First) (Photos 94–97)

94    Four Corners is a lengthy sequence composed of four separate movements, all similar but performed in different directions. Throughout, we will be using the diagonals so each movement finishes up facing a 'corner'.

To begin the first corner, sit back on your right leg and pivot on your left heel, to go slightly pigeon-toed. Allow your left hand to drop and drift to your centre, palm facing in and slightly upward.

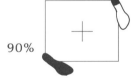

90%

*94 FOUR CORNERS (FIRST) Inbreath*

95    Relax the right elbow and let go of the Crane's Beak in your right hand. Bring your weight into the left foot and take a short step with the right, placing it down heel first, toes pointing west. Allow your centre to turn naturally towards the south-west as you do this. By now the left hand is almost 'cupping' the right elbow.

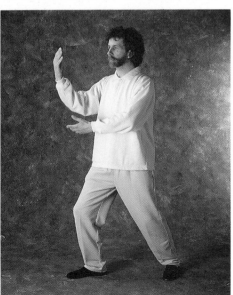

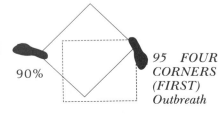

90%

*95 FOUR CORNERS (FIRST) Outbreath*

96    Raise the left foot and prepare to step out towards the south-west.

*Note:* before doing this, do make sure you sink strongly into your substantial leg. This will give you stability: a much-needed advantage when performing the movements that are to follow.

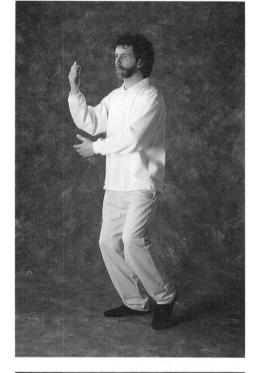

*96  FOUR CORNERS (FIRST) Inbreath*

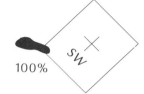

100%

97    Place the left foot down heel first, to the south-west, and as you bend the knee, spiral out with the hands so that the left hand rises up to about head height, while the right hand 'pushes' slightly upwards and forwards at about chest height. The right hand is central, in front of your chest, while the left hand is somewhat off of centre. Allow your waist to turn naturally towards your leading leg as the weight goes forward, head, hips and shoulders all facing south-west, left knee over left toes.

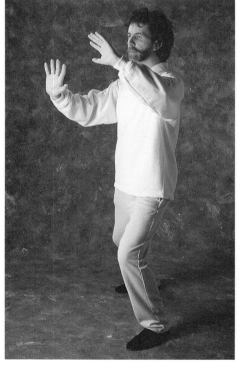

*97  FOUR CORNERS (FIRST) Outbreath*

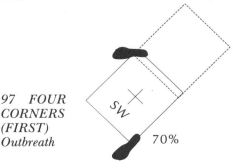

70%

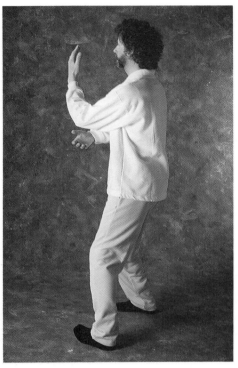

# Four Corners (Second) (Photos 98–101)

**98**   For the second corner we have to execute a large, three-quarters turn, clockwise, around to the south-east. To begin, transfer your weight to the rear leg; sit back and relax. Draw in your arms and turn the hands inwards. There are many variations on how the hands are placed at this point, but in the illustration my left palm is 'looking' at my left shoulder, with my right palm in the centre, tummy height, palm up – almost cupping the left elbow. At this point, with most of your weight in that rear leg, pivot on your left heel to get your left toes as far around to the north as is comfortable.

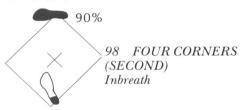

*98   FOUR CORNERS (SECOND) Inbreath*

**99**   Now transfer your weight into your left foot, sink into it and then pivot on the toes of your right foot, so that it too points in a northerly direction. This movement, and the others like it in the Four Corners sequence, are excellent for the ankles. It may take you some time to loosen up sufficiently to get these turns smooth, but it is well worth the effort. Don't forget those warm up exercises on page 12 to get the ankle joints loose before you start.

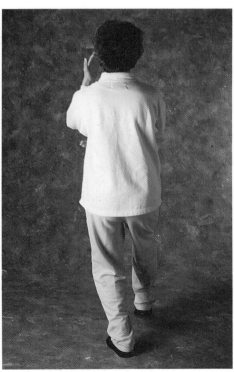

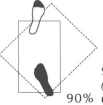

*99   FOUR CORNERS (SECOND) Outbreath*

100 With your weight now entirely in the left foot, start to think in terms of stepping towards the south-east by turning your eyes in that direction. Raise the right foot and turn the right hip out, ready to step with your right heel. Your palms at this stage are starting to think about spiralling outward as well.

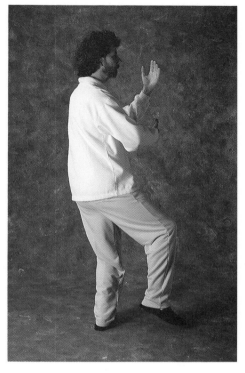

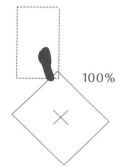

100% 

*100 FOUR CORNERS (SECOND) Inbreath*

101 Place the right foot down to the south-east, heel first, and bring your weight forward by bending the knee. Adjust the rear foot as soon as possible by pivoting on the heel, so that your back knee feels comfortable. At the same time spiral out with your hands, so that the right hand rises up to head height while the left hand 'pushes' slightly upwards and forwards at about chest height. The left hand is central, in front of your chest, while the right hand is somewhat off centre. Allow your waist to turn naturally towards your leading leg as the weight goes forward, head, hips and shoulders all facing south-east, right knee over right toes.

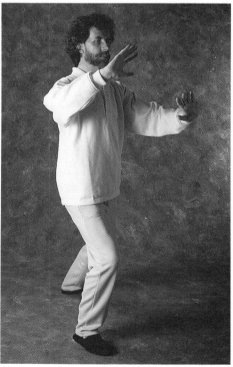

*101 FOUR CORNERS (SECOND) Outbreath*

SE

70%

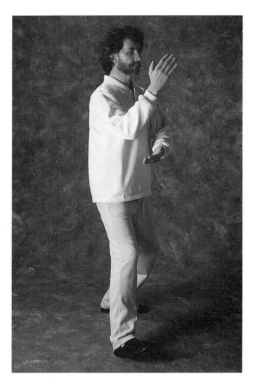

# Four Corners (Third) (Photos 102–105)

**102**   The stepping routine for the third corner is somewhat less complex. First of all, sit back onto the rear foot and relax the hands, letting them turn slightly inwards. The left hand begins to 'cup' the right elbow while the right hand 'looks' towards the left shoulder. Begin to raise the right foot and look towards the north-east.

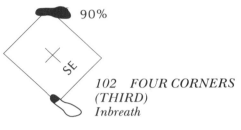

*102   FOUR CORNERS (THIRD) Inbreath*

**103**   Place the right foot down in front of your left foot. This might feel as if the right foot has stepped across the left, but in fact it is merely in front of it. Don't compress the groin area too much. Once done, slowly bring most of your weight into the right foot. This is a movement that helps work the inner aspect of the leg, especially if you keep your right foot pointed out. It is also beneficial for the hip joint. But don't strain, and make sure the feet are not too close together.

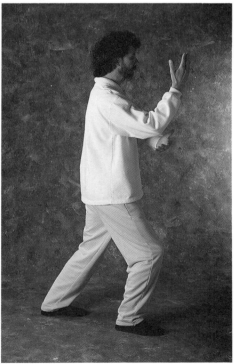

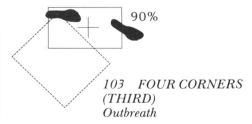

*103   FOUR CORNERS (THIRD) Outbreath*

104   With the next inhalation, raise the left foot and prepare to step with it towards the north-east. Sink entirely onto your right foot to do this.

*Note:* although the arms and elbows are fairly close in to your body at this point, do make sure – as always – that they are not touching the body. Keep a rounded aspect to the arms, even here, and allow the breath and the chi to move freely.

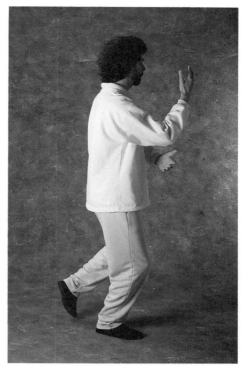

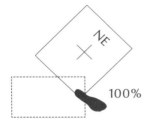

*104   FOUR CORNERS (THIRD) Inbreath*

100%

105   Continue by stepping out to the north-east with your left foot, heel first. Bring your weight forward by bending the left knee and make any necessary adjustment to the right heel. At the same time spiral out with the hands, lifting the left palm to about head height while pushing out and slightly upwards from the centre with your right palm at about chest height. The right hand is central, in front of your chest, while the left hand is somewhat off centre. Allow your waist to turn naturally towards your leading leg as the weight goes forward. Head, hips and shoulders all facing north-east, left knee over left toes.

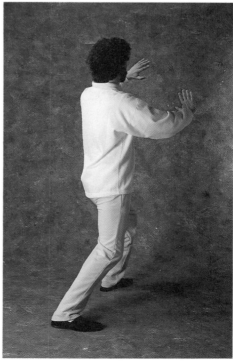

70%

*105   FOUR CORNERS (THIRD) Outbreath*

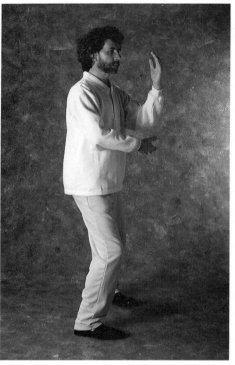

# Four Corners (Fourth) (Photos 106–109)

**106**  For your fourth and final corner, you have to take the long way around again for another three-quarters turn, clockwise to finish north-west. So once again, begin by sitting back onto your rear leg and relaxing the arms. Again, the hands turn inwards slightly as the right hand begins to 'cup' the left elbow, left palm looking in towards the right shoulder. Transfer your weight into your rear leg, then pivot on your left heel to get your left toes as far around to the south as is comfortable.

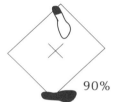

90%

*106   FOUR CORNERS (FOURTH) Inbreath*

**107**  Transfer your weight into your left foot, sink into it and then pivot on the toes of your right foot so that it too points in a southerly direction.

*Note:* movements such as you find here in Four Corners really encourage us to let go of tension in the lower abdomen and groin area, due to the constant opening up and directing of the hips, a place where energy often becomes congested through emotional or deep-seated psychological difficulties.

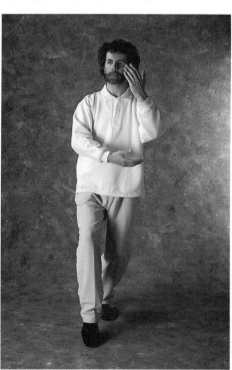

90%

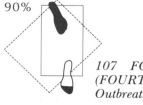

*107   FOUR CORNERS (FOURTH) Outbreath*

108    Breathe in and sink entirely into your left foot. Start to think in terms of stepping towards the north-west now, by turning your eyes in that direction. Raise the right foot and turn the right hip out, ready to step. Always test your balance before raising the foot – you have plenty of time with this manoeuvre.

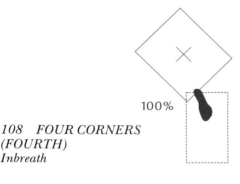

100%

*108   FOUR CORNERS*
*(FOURTH)*
*Inbreath*

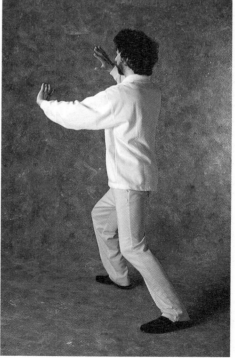

109    Now place the right foot down to the north-west, heel first, and bring your weight forward. Adjust the rear foot as soon as possible. At the same time, spiral out with your hands, lifting the right palm up to head height and pushing slightly forwards and upwards from the centre with the left palm, at about chest height. The left hand is central, in front of your chest, while the right hand is somewhat off centre. Allow your waist to turn naturally towards your leading leg as the weight goes forward. Head, hips and shoulders all face north-west, right knee over right toes.
    And that concludes the Four Corners sequence.

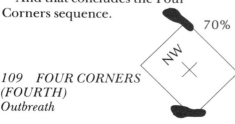

70%

NW

*109   FOUR CORNERS*
*(FOURTH)*
*Outbreath*

## Ward Off Left

After your fourth and final corner you simply step to the south with the right heel and do your Ward Off Left. We have met this movement before, of course, in Part One so refer to photo 10 to remind yourself of how this looks. The only difference is that you are coming into it from a slightly different direction this time, from the north-west rather than simply west, but it doesn't matter. Just relax the arms, sit back onto your left leg and pivot a little on your right heel to begin. Then shift your weight entirely into your right leg and step south. The rest is the same as described on page 24.

## Grasp Bird's Tail, Rollback, Press, Separate Hands and Push, Single Whip

After Ward Off Left, you continue with another Chorus, the final one in fact. Still exactly the same as shown in photos 11–23, it will bring you once again into a wide 70/30 stance, facing east (Single Whip).

## Snake Creeps Down

After your Chorus you simply repeat Snake Creeps Down, so refer to photos 71 and 72 to remind you of how this goes. Everything exactly the same. Breathe in at the top of the movement, then out as you squat down. Then let go of the Crane's Beak, come up, inhale, turn out the left toes and prepare for the next movement.

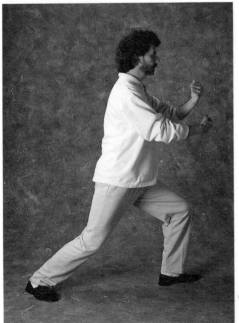

## Step Forward to Seven Stars (Photos 110–111)

110   With the left foot turned out to provide you with a broad base, raise the right foot and prepare to step forward into a narrow toe stance towards the east. Your hands are drawn up in front of you and your right hand is just beginning to form itself into a loose fist.

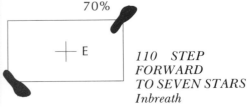

*110   STEP FORWARD TO SEVEN STARS*
Inbreath

111  Make loose fists now with both hands and complete your narrow toe stance with the right foot. As you go, allow the wrists to cross, left wrist resting on top of the right, and rotate them so that the knuckle side of the hands are turned towards you. This rolling motion of the wrists feels particularly good, as it accompanies the upward and forward movement of the body. It is as if your entire body energy is being focused in that small rotation at the end.

*111  STEP FORWARD TO SEVEN STARS*
*Outbreath*

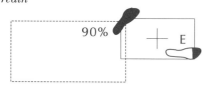

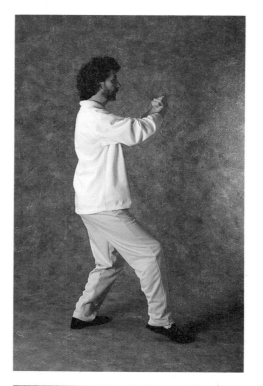

## Step Back to Ride The Tiger (Photos 112–113)

112  Step back with your right toes. Then bring all your weight into the right foot and settle down. While this is happening, your hands separate and the right hand, after dropping a little, spirals out around in a wide arc to the side of the head in a movement that looks, just for an instant, a little like Crane Spreads Its Wings. The left hand, meanwhile, lowers diagonally to a position just left of centre, hip height. As the weight sinks into the right foot, straighten the left foot by raising it very slightly to settle back down into a narrow toe stance, facing due east. All this is accomplished with the inhalation.

*112  STEP BACK TO RIDE THE TIGER*
*Inbreath*

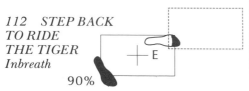

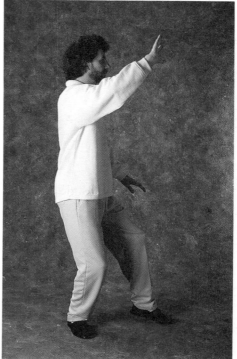

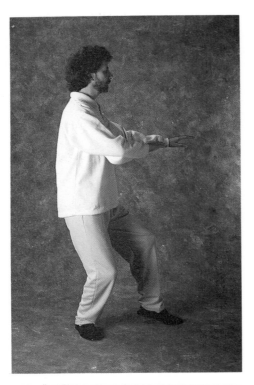

113   Keep that right hand moving, swooping back down in a wide diagonal arc towards your left hip where the left hand just rises slightly in response to meet it. Turn your waist slightly anti-clockwise as you do this and really let that right hand *soar*, so that as it comes across and down, you should be able to see the back of the hand. The result is a really good, free twist to the joints of the arm.

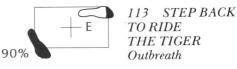

90%

*113   STEP BACK TO RIDE THE TIGER*
*Outbreath*

## Sweep The Lotus (Photos 114–115)

114   Here, you are going to turn the body right around through 360°, with the left leg sweeping half of the way round off the ground. Prepare for this movement by sinking strongly into the right foot, then raise the left foot and straighten the leg somewhat. Next sweep the left foot around, south through to west, close to the ground and using the momentum of your arms and waist as the whole body turns counter-clockwise on the ball of your right foot. This inevitably has to be done fairly quickly, especially when you are learning, but it is surprising how graceful you can make it in time. Touch down to the west with the heel of your right foot.

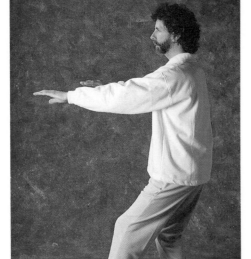

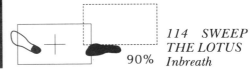

90%

*114   SWEEP THE LOTUS*
*Inbreath*

115    To complete the next 180°, use a combination of pivoting on heels and toes. Sources differ as to precisely how this should be achieved. Some people use left heel and right toes, others the complete reverse! The best thing is to do whatever seems comfortable to you. Providing you have executed the first half of the circle smoothly, with a graceful sweeping action of the left foot close to the ground, the rest is not so critical. Eventually, you will be back facing east, the arms still parallel to the ground and the right foot ahead of your left. Sink onto the rear leg and prepare for a kick.

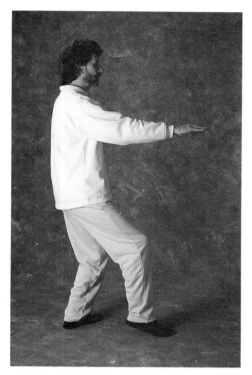

100%

*115    SWEEP*
*THE LOTUS*
*Inbreath finishes*

## Crescent Kick (Photo 116)

116    Allow the arms to drift a little to the right of centre and then set up your kick by sinking totally into the left foot. This is an unusual style of kick. Were you to be actually making contact with anything, it would be the outer edge of your right foot that would do so. This is because the hip directs the leg outwards in a great arc. But first, as with all kicks, you need to bring up the knee. Then the rest of the leg extends as you sweep out with it to the right. As this occurs, your arms return to the centre, travelling in the opposite direction.

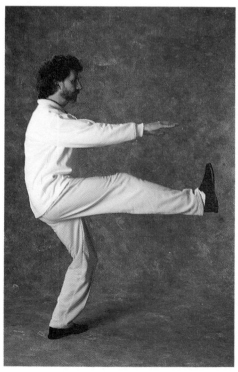

100%

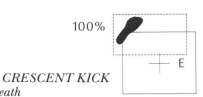

*116    CRESCENT KICK*
*Outbreath*

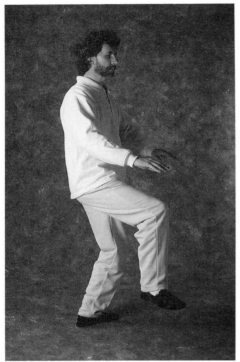

# Sink Down and Brush Knee (Photos 117–118)

117 This is not a classical tai chi movement as such and is sadly often rushed. I consider it to be important, however, since it encourages relaxation following what is a particularly dynamic movement. Firstly, drop the shin and relax the wrists. This should be accompanied by an inhalation, the foot remaining in the air. If you feel you may have lost your 'root' temporarily during the Crescent Kick, this is an excellent opportunity to re-establish it.

100%

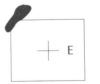

*117 SINK DOWN AND BRUSH KNEE Inbreath*

118 With the next exhalation, place the right foot down with the toes pointing outwards. Allow the arms to brush the right knee a little as you do this and bring most of your weight forward by bending the right knee. Let your centre follow, slightly clockwise, as you do this. Relax the shoulders. Try to imagine an energy connection between your palms and the ground. Sink, sink, sink. Find your roots.

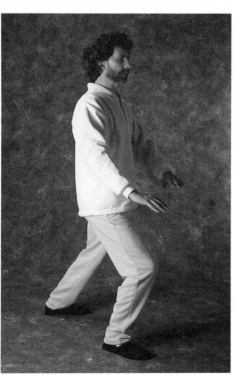

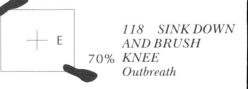

70%

*118 SINK DOWN AND BRUSH KNEE Outbreath*

# Bend The Bow and Shoot The Tiger (Photos 119–120)

119   Imagine a long staff or bow which you clasp with your hands. In other words make two loose fists quite low down over your right thigh. Then, with the knuckles of the right hand turned inwards, bring the right fist up in a graceful arc to about head height and centred, as if thrusting one end of the bow into the ground.

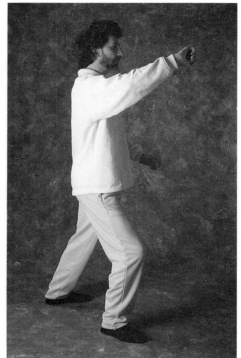

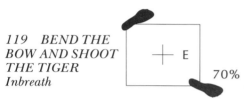

*119   BEND THE BOW AND SHOOT THE TIGER*
*Inbreath*

E

70%

120   The right hand then comes back a little, closer to your head, while the left fist separates outwards and forwards at about abdomen height. The weight comes forward entirely after this, so that the back foot actually leaves the ground momentarily as the waist turns to accommodate the arm movements. Bring the foot through, alongside your right foot if you wish, but don't overdo this. This is a movement which can easily lead to a lopsided appearance or to raised or tense shoulders. It is important, therefore, to monitor your actions closely to make sure the shoulders do not come up – especially the right side. Keep them level.

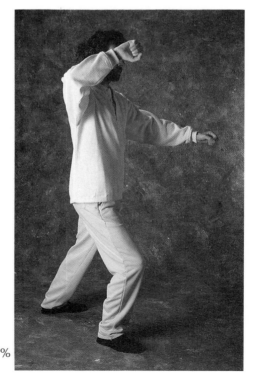

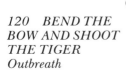

*120   BEND THE BOW AND SHOOT THE TIGER*
*Outbreath*

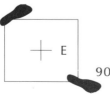

E

90%

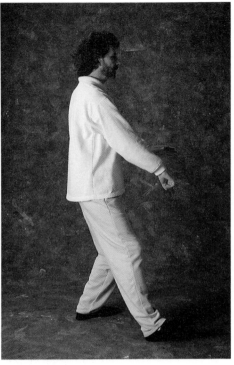

# Step Forward, Parry and Punch (Photos 121–124)

**121**   We have met with this sequence before, at the very end of Part One. We use it again here to close the whole form – the only difference being that in Part One the whole thing began from a Brush Knee and Push position with the left leg forward whereas here, of course, we begin with the right leg forward. From the previous movement, it is assumed that you have already put back that left foot firmly on the ground. As this occurs, lower the arms and let go of the left fist. Simultaneously, spiral down to the left hip with your right fist and allow your weight to flow into the left foot.

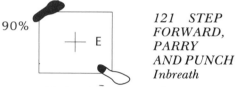

90%

*121   STEP FORWARD, PARRY AND PUNCH Inbreath*

**122**   Lift the right foot and turn out the toes so that as you put it back down again, more or less in the same spot, it will point out at a good wide angle, nearly south in fact. Bend the right knee and bring your weight forward. At the same time 'throw' the fist over to your right hip, palm side up in readiness to punch. The waist will naturally want to turn slighly clockwise as you do this. Keep the left hand low and relaxed but – as before – if you feel it wants to follow the right palm, more to the centre of your body then let it do so.

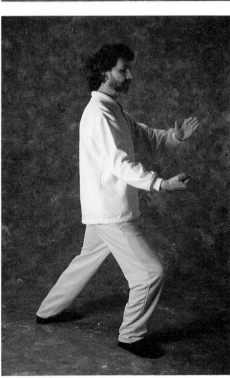

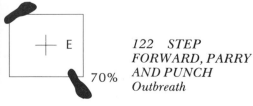

70%

*122   STEP FORWARD, PARRY AND PUNCH Outbreath*

123    Raise your left foot and begin to step forward. Keep the left hand relaxed and the fist in readiness at your right hip. As you go, try drawing in the left toes a little towards the right heel before stepping out to the east. As with the previous Step Forward, Parry and Punch sequence concluding Part One, it is useful to get those right toes out at a generous angle. That way you will be able to pivot on the heel and your centre will be able to 'rotate' into the movement that follows.

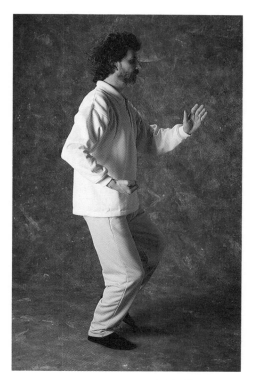

*123    STEP FORWARD, PARRY AND PUNCH*
*Inbreath*

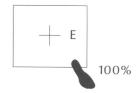

100%

124    Now place the left heel down and bend the left knee, the foot facing directly east. Just as this occurs, or perhaps just a fraction before, you 'parry' with your left arm or, in other words, raise the forearm to a near vertical position as if deflecting an oncoming force. Then punch very slowly towards the east. This is now precisely the same as the previous parry and punch and if in any doubt, refer back to the instructions accompanying photo 37. Remember that half-turn of the fist that goes with the punch.

*124    STEP FORWARD, PARRY AND PUNCH*
*Outbreath*

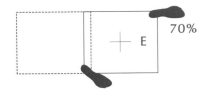

70%

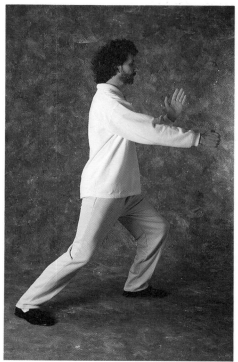

## Release Arm and Push

**Refer to photos 38–40 for this sequence.**

## Close The Form

After **Release Arm and Push**, you simply turn back to the south and close the whole form – just as you finished Part One. This concluding sequence is illustrated here again for your convenience.

If you have done everything correctly, your feet should finish up in more or less the same place from which you started, emphasising the cyclic nature of the tai chi form. Here, at the finish, take a moment just to relax, keeping your shoulder-width stance. Experience how the body feels. Imagine your feet putting roots down, way into the ground, and try to keep in touch still with the feeling of being suspended from above, with the spine straight and yet perfectly relaxed. Take a few deep breaths into the abdomen.

> 66 *Winning has to do with nothing other than feeling good about yourself.* 99
>
> E.M. Hass

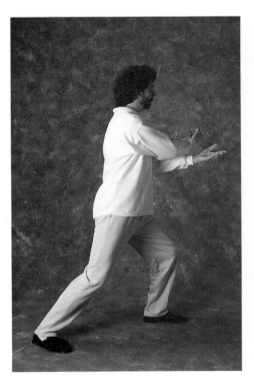 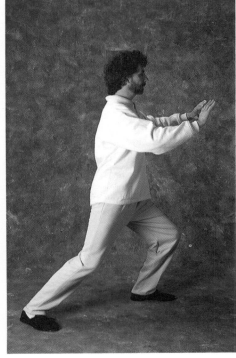

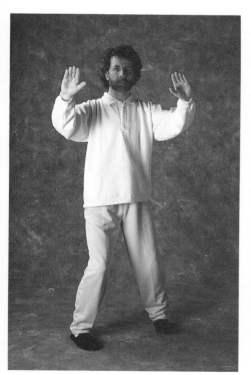
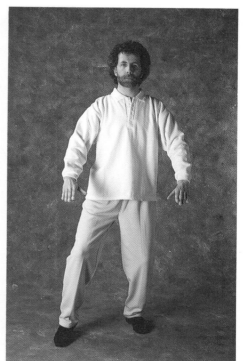
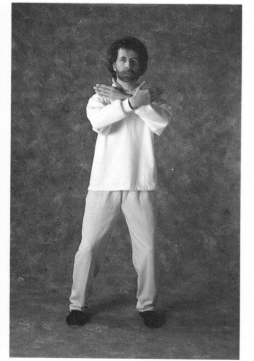
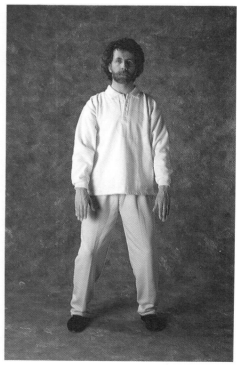

# 6

## GOING FURTHER

## Additional notes on some of the movements

### Opening

The even distribution of weight here between the two feet rarely occurs in the form. It is not considered a strong position. You'll find it at the beginning and again at the end.

The opening sequence is, of course, a relatively simple kind of movement but it contains many important principles. For example, keeping the shoulders relaxed as you raise your arms is vital. Think, too, of the way the breathing is reflected in the upward and downward, forward and backward movements of the arms and hands: Yang and Yin right here at the very start. Also, here at the beginning you encounter the typical pattern of stepping – that is, shifting your weight to what is to become the 'substantial' leg, then stepping out with the empty foot and finally adjusting the other foot to complete the movement (photos 1 and 2). This pattern of *1. Empty, 2. Step and 3. Adjust* is the basis of almost every movement you will encounter in this or any other tai chi form.

### Turn Right

If you can get your right toes 90° from your left heel, as shown in the foot diagram, great! But don't worry if you can't. Some people may feel their left knee tensing up if they go all the way and to keep on doing this would simply be counter-productive. As with all these movements, particularly during the early days when your body is accustoming itself to their demands, a little at a time is best.

### Ward Off Left

This is a strong position. Great tai chi masters use it to demonstrate the essence of being rooted – with several hapless students lined up and pushing with all their might against the master's arm, unable to budge him at all. Surprisingly, most of us, with a little practice, can achieve something similar, albeit on a considerably more modest scale. Try it with

just one partner pushing against your arm. Experiment by moving your
feet until you feel the pressure being transferred away and into the
ground.

## Grasp Bird's Tail

We are at this point immersed in a whole set of movements which
traditionally have the prefix of Grasp Bird's Tail or sometimes Grasp
Sparrow's Tail. This one, for instance, is Grasp Bird's Tail Ward Off
Right, while the previous movement and also those of Rollback and Press
which follow are all similarly prefixed with the Bird's Tail title – all of
which can be decidedly confusing. In my classes, therefore, I usually
reserve the term Grasp Bird's Tail for this one movement only, since it
most typifies the action of somebody holding the bird's neck with the
right hand while the left hand smooths the long plumage of the bird's
tail.

## Rollback

This is one of the few Yin movements to actually have a name. Like all
Yin parts of the form, Rollback is only the duration of an inbreath but
don't rush it. It is a beautiful movement to perform, with a great feeling
of energy returning inwards. Allow the hands to roll gently, the left palm
almost sliding down the right forearm, all the while the weight shifting
slowly backwards.

## Press

Although when you see this movement being performed it looks as if the
hands and arms are doing a lot of work, in fact they do not move all that
much. Most of the movement is created by the turning of the waist, firstly
towards the south, then back to the west again. Relax the arms and just let
them follow the movements of the body.

## Separate Hands and Push

A common error at the start of this movement is to lean too far back, as if
recoiling from something in shock. It can look quite comical. Make sure
you are not doing this. Use a mirror if necessary and check that the spine
remains vertical, like a plumb line suspended from above.

*Note:* everything from Grasp Bird's Tail through to Push is done with
both feet planted firmly on the ground. Try to resist any temptation to
raise the right toes as you shift your weight back. It is surprising how
many students find this difficult and short of actually nailing one's boots
to the floor, the only way to eliminate this is through continuous practice
and self-observation – and also perhaps trying to loosen and massage
your knees and ankles regularly to eliminate tension in those places.

# Single Whip

Regarding the pigeon-toed stance used during the early parts of this movement, there are many reasons why you should persevere with this. It encourages the rooting of the feet and teaches you to keep the knees apart when the weight moves from side to side. So keep trying until it starts to feel good.

Regarding photos 19 and 20, the right forearm moves back across horizontally, the elbow pointing west. In contrast, however, the left hand should swoop down in a graceful arc to your right hip. For this, it may help to imagine a barrow full of sand – scoop up the sand. Then, as the hand lifts and spirals out to the east to complete the movement (photos 22 and 23), you are permitting the sand to trickle slowly from your hand. As this occurs, the feeling can be one of release, like setting free a coiled up spring – a very expansive, Yang type of movement. Enjoy it.

At the very end, the shape formed by the left arm and hand should be a relaxed one. In profile it looks a bit like the spout of an old-fashioned teapot. No tension in the wrist, elbows or fingers, please. Let the arms 'float'.

# Play Guitar

Those musicians among you who do actually play a guitar will have realised by now that this movement bears absolutely no resemblance whatsoever to the actions of playing a real guitar. Something has undoubtedly got lost in translation from the original Chinese name for this movement. There is, I believe, a Chinese instrument which, when played with a bow, would accommodate arm movements of this kind but it is certainly not a guitar.

# Pull and Step With Shoulder

A common error at the end of this movement is that as the body rotates anti-clockwise, it tends to lean forward as well. The result is a rather uncomfortable, twisted-up appearance which will impede the flow of chi. Again, always think of the plumb line and keep that spine straight! Incidentally, although the body is turned to the south-east at the end of this movement, the eyes continue to look south. This provides an opportunity to exercise the eye muscles as well as everything else. Nothing is wasted in tai chi.

# Crane Spreads Its Wings

The crane has always been an important and much celebrated creature in oriental culture and mythology, combining two great qualities that people from all ages have always admired – namely strength but also gracefulness. The execution of this movement – a favourite among many who practise tai chi – is often a visible indication as to how far the student has managed to integrate these two often opposing qualities in his or her life.

*Note:* although at the beginning of this movement, the left hand appears not to be doing much, do not on that account let it hang lifeless at your side. Your hands and your feet are never entirely empty in tai chi. Always bear in mind the Tai Chi T'u symbol and the tiny seed of Yang that you find deep within the Yin, ready to transform itself into something greater.

## Brush Left Knee and Push

There is lots happening all at once with this movement. One of my teachers once likened it to a children's game in which you are urged to try patting your head and rubbing your stomach all at the same time. It requires great co-ordination. But then this is precisely one of the things you are seeking to develop with your tai chi, so stick with it. Incidentally, you can turn to photo 87, where the same movement is repeated facing west, to see how this looks from the other side. Note how the left hand remains hovering somewhat over the left thigh. Don't let it fall away behind you.

## Step Forward, Parry and Punch

The tai chi fist is soft, loosely held, not tightly clenched. There is no anger in this kind of fist and it does not punch. Rather, it is a demonstration of will and self-confidence. Ideally, the thumb and the first joint of the index finger should be in contact. Those who do yoga will recognise this – a *mudra* – as a means of concentrating energy.

During the forward stepping sequence (see photos 35–36) it is acceptable to keep the left arm low and relaxed. I believe this is the way Cheng Man Ching taught the movement during his latter years. However, if you feel it wants to follow the right hand somewhat, across to the centre of your body for instance, then let it do so. Some people move it in a great arc from behind the left side over to the centre (as in the traditional long form), but this is not necessary in the context of the kind of tai chi being demonstrated here.

With the punch itself, your fist makes one half-turn as it goes, so that whereas it started off with the palm side up, it turns in mid-flight so that by the end you have the thumb edge facing upwards. Finally, if you can, do pivot a little on the heel of the right foot so that the whole body 'twists' into the movement as your weight carries the punch forward.

## Diagonal Chorus (Rollback, Press, Separate Hands and Push, and Single Whip)

There are two main reasons why we bother with the added complication of the diagonal axis. The first is an historic one, in deference to the Taoist world picture of nine directions – i.e. the four compass points, the four intermediate points and centre. This is set out in the *I Ching* or Book of Changes. Each of the points has a philosophical correlation and in one of the oldest arrangements, the north-west is the direction of 'The Mountain', of late autumn, rest and keeping still.

The second reason is wholly practical. Up to now you have been able to use your surroundings to orient yourself – using the walls of the room, maybe, to line up your feet. Now you are forced to orient yourself entirely by reference to your own centre. This increased self-awareness and the ability to sense one's own boundaries clearly is of great value.

With this first repetition of the Chorus, you add a really big chunk onto your form without having to learn very much new. However, while you are getting used to the diagonals, do please check your feet and be honest: are you still managing to retain your shoulder-width stance? Tai chi is always testing you. The moment you feel you are getting along just wonderfully and your ego starts to soar, something is thrown in your path – a challenge, of course, not an obstacle – for you to overcome. The diagonal axis is just one such challenge.

## Repulse Monkey

Although the foot diagrams indicate a wide stance, you will in practice probably find yourself stepping back fairly narrow. This is all right as long as it is not so excessively narrow that you are unstable. Cheng Man Ching actually advocated stepping back with the feet parallel – which is not at all easy for beginners – but why not give it a try! Also, with each step back and as the hand comes down to waist height, make sure you keep your elbow well out from your side. It's a bit like having a rolled-up blanket under your arm – really that much space between ribs and elbows. Allow yourself to breathe.

The Repulse Monkey sequence should be performed with plenty of body movement – turn the waist each time to accommodate the generous back swing of the arm, thereby emulating the actions of a real monkey swinging through the branches. Keep your wrists relaxed at all times – again, just like the monkey. Also, allow your eyes to follow the palm each time as it circles back. The monkey will not come to seize the food if he thinks you are looking at him so divert your gaze to the palm instead as it moves behind your shoulder. Do remember, however, that this has to be achieved without excessive movement of the head in relation to the shoulders. Just turn the waist and use the eyes. They will benefit greatly from this gentle exercise.

## Diagonal Flying

In keeping with the imagery of the monkey in our little story, here you could say you are picking up the monkey and putting him back on the tree. The right hand with its upward-facing palm does tend to have the appearance of 'offering up'. Also, the whole movement is like a spring coiling and expanding, similar in feeling to the Single Whip, i.e. progressive contraction (Yin) transforming into its opposite, expansion (Yang). A good movement for strengthening the waist and for helping to remove congestion from the abdomen and chest.

# Cloudy Hands

When you step inwards with the right foot (photo 62) place it down *no closer* than shoulder width to your left foot. A common error here is to step in too close, so you start to wobble. The success of this manoeuvre depends largely on having sufficient width to play with initially, which means that when we draw up the left foot in photo 58, we make it at a distance of at least one and a half shoulder-widths from the right.

Always step just a fraction prior to changing the hands. As always, the movements of the arms reflect those of the waist and centre of the body. As it turns, the hands follow, rather than the other way around. Keep in mind the phrase 'step and change – step and change' to keep the correct order. If you can manage to keep that parallel aspect of the feet, you will find that every joint in the body receives a gentle movement and internal 'massage' – the toes, ankles, knees and hips, spine, shoulders, elbows and fingers all getting worked. It does, however, require rather a lot of co-ordination and practice to perform happily and at first it may seem as if the brain is getting its fair share of arduous work as well. So here are a few tips to help you remember things.

In Cloudy Hands, always turn your waist in the direction of your highest arm. Then, just prior to changing the hands, step with the opposite leg to which you have turned. Although during the learning phase, all these movements are made in a rather precise fashion, you will eventually free up quite a bit and start to flow. To help, here are a couple of rather mixed metaphors to assist you with the actions of the hands. Think of the upper hand 'stroking' downwards, as if along the nose of a pony or furry creature of some kind. *Softly.* Meanwhile, think of the lower hand as having its fingers stuck in a pot of sticky stuff, glue or honey. Imagine the sticky strands coming up, adhering slightly to your fingers as you go.

Peculiar as all this may well sound, it encourages a certain softness in the hands and is often a great help to those wishing to deepen their understanding of the movements. For the time being, however, make sure you follow the instructions for the hands very closely.

# Snake Creeps Down

Most western students find this a particularly difficult manoeuvre to perform, basically because they try too hard. Unless you train and stretch yourself constantly every day you are unlikely to achieve the kind of standard that Chinese masters display. Do not try to sink down too far, therefore. It is not necessary to do this in order to gain the benefits from the movement. What is important is as follows:

**1** Try to retain as straight a back as possible – don't lean over just in order to get yourself down a few inches lower. The gentle bearing down of your rib cage upon your liver as you sink down is very helpful, the liver being a vital organ that performs around 500 different chemical functions for us, often simultaneously.

**2** Do make sure you turn in your left toes as you sink down and then turn them straight again as your hand sweeps forward. This stimulates several important acu-points in the inside heel that are related to your Kidney chi.

**3** Finally, make sure your weight remains in your right foot throughout. Even as your hand sweeps forward, keep the weight back. The right knee should remain directly above the right heel to achieve this.

## Golden Pheasant

The essence of this sequence is that of a smooth interchange and transference of weight and energy. Therefore, it is not simply a case of bringing one side down and then the other side up. Finish the first side off properly by sinking clearly into the right leg before raising the left. Also remember the Tai Chi T'u symbol and keep a little bit of energy in the less active hand. Don't let it hang lifeless while you're busy with the other side. Instead, imagine an energy connection between your lowest palm and the ground. The fingers of the raised hand, meanwhile, are close together, though not tense. Keep your eyes focused ahead; don't look down. That will help you to balance. Finally, *keep it loose* – don't crease up or hunch your shoulders and only raise the knee as far as is comfortable. Realise your limitations and be confident that, bit by bit, your balance will improve.

## Pat The Horse (Left and Right)

Despite the name of this movement, *do not pat*. This is not what is taking place. Rather, you should be stroking across gently with the palm, fingers very relaxed.

*Note:* regarding Pat The Horse on the Left, this is not simply a mirror image of Pat The Horse on the Right. In both instances, it is your right leg which is slightly forward of the left at the finish and in both instances you turn your centre towards the leading leg, i.e. slightly clockwise as you pat the horse.

## Kick With Toes (Left and Right)

The separation of the hands precedes the kick; never perform these actions together, as this would simply dissipate the energy into too many limbs at once. It is also worth remembering that toe kicks are really just an extension of movements featuring narrow toe stances – like Crane Spreads Its Wings – and you should feel no less certain of your footing on one than on the other. In both cases, you are aiming for a gentle stimulation and stretch along the front aspect of the leg, thereby encouraging the flow of energy in the Stomach and Spleen acu-channels that are situated there. This is beneficial for many internal functions related to digestion and the assimilation and use of liquids.

# Turn and Kick With Sole

To kick with the sole or the heel of a foot, you naturally tend to point the toes upwards. This stimulates an entirely different set of acu-channels in the leg to those activated by the toe kicks. Here, as with the narrow heel stances of the form, it is the posterior aspect of the leg, the hamstrings and Achilles tendon, that get the work. Equally importantly, however, these movements tend to stimulate the Kidney and Bladder acu-channels of the body. This is beneficial for all things connected to the reproductive organs, the urinary system and also the skeletal system and bone marrow.

# All Brush Knee and Pushes

All the expansive, backward circling movements serve to naturally open up the chest area, where many of the acu-channels either begin or end. Equally as important, the vital lymph glands situated in the chest, throat and armpits get massaged. The lymph fluid rids the body of poisons and provides defences against disease and infection. With the decreasing efficiency of our immune responses these days – largely a result of atmospheric pollution and abnormal level of ultraviolet radiation reaching the Earth's surface – exercises of this kind cannot be too highly recommended.

# Brush Knee and Punch Low

As with the previous instance in which you delivered a 'punch', here the fist does one half-turn in midflight. The only difference is that here it is the knuckle side of the fist facing upwards to begin with, whereas before it was the palm side turned up. This variation is due to the difference in height to which the fist is to be projected and ensures a fluid action which greatly benefits the joints of the wrist and arm.

# Four Corners

This elegant sequence is sometimes called Fair Lady Works At Shuttles, because the movements of the hands are thought to mimic somewhat the actions of someone weaving and using a shuttle. Whether this is entirely accurate or not is of little importance, for the name itself does intimate the soft, delicate nature of the actions in which the hands alternate quite noticeably between expanding and contracting aspects. Allow your hands to become Yin as you turn, then Yang as you spiral out with the arms at the end of each corner. Think, too, of a flower closing in and opening out alternately.

Here are some 'rules' which will help you to learn and remember the sequence.

**1** At the beginning of each corner, as you start to turn, simply use the lowest hand to cup the opposite elbow. It is amazing how many students make hard work of this manoeuvre by reversing the hands. Just keep the upper hand up and the lower hand low, then sit back, cup the elbow and commence your turn.

**2**  At the conclusion of each corner, the side with the leading leg always has the highest arm.

**3**  With corners One, Two and Four, always use a combination of turning on your left heel and right toes, plus of course a large step round at the end.

## Step Forward to Seven Stars

The 'seven stars' referred to here make up the constellation of Ursa Major – the Big Dipper or Great Bear. If you look at the Big Dipper on a winter's evening you will see it with the tail end downwards. The tai chi movement described here tends to look a bit similar in profile – the leg being the tail, the arms forming the bowl shape above it.

## Step Back to Ride The Tiger

At this stage of your tai chi training it is assumed that you will be able to recognise and eliminate tension if and when it occurs and here, with the raising of the right arm and the turning of the wrist joint, you must be especially vigilant. The part played by the left arm in this action should not be neglected, either. Remember the Tai Chi T'u and the energy seed always present, even in the most Yin places. Think of two friends – the right hand makes a long journey to visit the left hand, but out of courtesy the left hand makes a little trip too, just to the garden gate, to meet the other. It is this natural 'etiquette' of the tai chi movements, in which one limb is very often echoing slightly the actions of the other, that helps to ensure the Yin/Yang balance of your form.

Incidentally the tiger, which crops up frequently in the names of the movements, is a symbol, in part, for the chi. In the west we have known this as 'animal magnetism', of course. One of the images associated with this movement is of a sleeping tiger, resting on the ground. As you step back you place your right foot on his back and the left foot, very gingerly, upon his neck. When he wakes up – as it might be presumed a tiger would most likely do with somebody on its back – the idea is that your balance is so excellent with all your tai chi training that you can simply ride him, no matter how much he tries to shake you off. It is not, however, recommended that you put this into practice.

## Sweep The Lotus

Like the previous turn on one leg (photos 84–85) this is another one of those tai chi movements best not learned too close to any precious antiques or porcelain. Don't panic with it! When some beginners first see this movement, they mistakenly believe the entire 360° turn is enacted in one go. As you have seen, this is not the case. Just concentrate initially on the first half of the turn, with the left foot above the ground. Thereafter, use both feet to complete the circle.

*Note:* it is important to make sure the forearms remain parallel to the ground during your turn. Try not to flail out too much with the hands as you go and that way you'll feel good about the movement. Sink, sink, sink and your balance will improve every time.

# Crescent Kick

This type of movement where the arms and leg travel in different directions can be beneficial for the spine, helping to relieve congestion in the acu-channels that surround it. However, if you do have a particularly bad back or are prone to disc trouble, it would be best to treat this movement with caution until your back has healed.

*Note:* this movement is also sometimes called the Lotus Kick. The symbolism of the lotus here and in the preceding movement is rather obscure but I was once told it referred to a lotus flower on the surface of a pool. The sweeping of the lotus is therefore the removal of the flower, without presumably getting one's feet wet. This is perhaps not as peculiar as it sounds, since it encourages us to keep the foot close to the ground during the turn. Another version tells us of the lotus flower with its round petals that seem to rotate in the wind, thereby inspiring the pattern of circular movements and the swirling kick featured here.

# Bend The Bow and Shoot The Tiger

The idea of the bow here is a good one. If you imagine a flexible bow, held in your hands, it ensures the correct alignment of the two fists. Observe your hands during this sequence and make certain that they could, theoretically, always be holding a bow or rod of some kind. The bow can bend a little but it must never snap. Initially, the bow itself is picked up in a horizontal position (photo 119), but then it goes near vertical as the fists separate (photo 120). Whatever happens, however, always keep the hollow part of the fists aligned, clasping the bow.

And with that, we come to the end of the instruction section of this book. Although you have now learned the movements in a basic sense, this is actually just the beginning of your tai chi studies. In the next chapters we will explore ways in which you can deepen your understanding of the subject and enhance your experience of chi.

> 66 *Perseverance is one of the fundamental requirements in practising T'ai-chi Ch'uan. No results can be obtained without it.* 99
>
> Yearning K. Chen

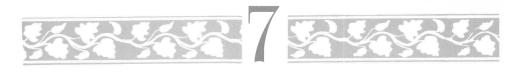

# TAI CHI AND HEALTH

Unlike traditional oriental medicine, with its well-documented network of therapeutic points and channels, the movements of tai chi have often been a source for speculation on precisely what benefits they bring in terms of health. Yet everyone involved with the subject would agree that regular practice is effective in promoting, restoring and maintaining the body's natural vitality and well-being. How precisely this happens is not always known. In this chapter I will list those correlations that I am aware of, taken from a variety of sources, and will also include my own observations based on the teachings of Traditional Chinese Medicine – TCM.

## Blood supply

Because of the emphasis on calm regular breathing and on practice in the open air, when possible, regular tai chi will inevitably assist the body's circulatory system. The extensive use of leg muscles stimulates the return flow of venous blood to the heart and lungs, while the relaxed focus of muscles in the upper body promotes an efficient supply of blood to all the major organs, to the brain and to the joints. Moreover, after an eight-minute form at a fairly low level of stance (slightly lower than that illustrated in this book) the heart rate increases gradually to a level consistent with the demands of moderate fitness training. This in turn helps to regulate blood pressure.

There are no special movements in the tai chi form that relate to the vascular system more than any other function of the body, but all heel stances and heel kicks stimulate the calf muscles, assisting circulation, and Crane Spreads Its Wings may also be helpful, since it gently stretches and brings out the heart channel in the arms. Also, the constant movement of the ankle joints throughout the form stimulates important points on the Spleen, Liver and Kidney acu-channels, while that of the wrists and forearms stimulates the Heart and Pericardium channels – all of which adds to the efficiency of the circulation and the strength of the blood vessels themselves. The kidneys are also partly responsible for maintenance of correct blood pressure in terms of western physiology so the benefits tend to dovetail nicely.

# Breathing

Tai chi has enormous benefits for the lungs. The continued expanding and contracting movements of the form massage and stimulate the lungs, helping them to take in lifegiving oxygen and to eliminate waste gases from the blood stream. The originator of the short Yang form, Cheng Man Ching, suffered from tuberculosis as a young man and the prognosis for his recovery was not good. Tai chi not only helped him overcome his illness, it also gave him enormous strength in later life.

With a good supply of oxygen, all the organs and systems of the body are able to function well. Oxygen helps us to maintain a suitable body weight as well, since it is essential for the burning of calories. Slimmers take note, you need to assist the process by looking after your lungs.

Parts of the form which are particularly beneficial for the lungs are the Pushes and Ward Off movements along with Grasp Bird's Tail and Press.

# Lymph

The lymph is a much neglected and little understood substance. Most people are familiar with the heart and the circulation of blood in the body but the existence of an internal cleansing medium, which helps us to fight off disease and to rid the body of toxins and waste products, is generally not so well known. We usually hear about the lymph nodes – places where the lymph fluid concentrates – when they become enlarged during illness. Yet they are constantly at work for us, keeping us well.

The lymph fluid, however, does not have a pump, like the blood has the heart, to move it around the body. It relies on physical movement instead, exercise and so on; the gentle, expansive, non-tensile movements of tai chi are ideal in this respect. Moreover, because most of the major lymph glands are situated in the chest, throat, armpits, groin, elbows and knees, it would seem that these are expressly targeted by many of the movements found in the form: all those that open up the chest area, for instance, such as Repulse Monkey or Brush Knee and Push; or those that free up the groin through expansive turning movements, such as Diagonal Flying and Four Corners; and finally, all those heel kicks and narrow heel stances to stimulate the rear aspect of the knee.

> 66 *T'ai-chi Ch'uan is closely related to Meditation. Long practice of Meditation may hinder blood circulation, but T'ai-chi Ch'uan helps to quicken it. It also helps to bring about the peace of mind and the exercise of breathing as desired by practisers of Meditation.* 99
>
> Yearning K. Chen

# Nerves, sensations and thought

The autonomic nervous system, that part of our body-intelligence that works independently of consciousness, is generally classified into two parts, the sympathetic and the parasympathetic. The former works mainly to prepare the body for action, increasing heartbeat, suspending digestive processes and carrying out a thousand other functions of which we are not consciously aware, while the latter prepares the body for rest so that it can recover from vigorous activity.

Clearly, then, tai chi would benefit the parasympathetic enormously, while also helping us to relax and cope with stress, anxiety and insomnia. But tai chi also works on the entire central nervous system through movements which stimulate and increase flexibility in the spinal cord such as Crane Spreads Its Wings, Golden Pheasant and Repulse Monkey. Meanwhile, the characteristically erect spine of tai chi encourages the free flow of cerebrospinal fluid, helping to relieve pressure on the intervertebral discs and spinal nerves.

The cerebrospinal fluid itself is an amazing substance. Through research in the exciting new field of craniosacral osteopathy, a very subtle rhythm has been located – called the 'cranial rhythmic impulse' – in which not only the cerebrospinal fluid but also all the membranes enveloping every organ, muscle, nerve and blood vessel throughout the human body beat gently in synchronisation. The entire body, therefore, is constantly responding to a basic tempo that originates within the central nervous system itself. Even the joints of the skull and sacrum resonate to it in a subtle way that can be detected through the fingers and palms of the experienced craniosacral practitioner.

But the astonishing thing for us, in the world of tai chi, is that this rhythm, generally around 12 to 14 beats per minute, is precisely that at which the tai chi form is enacted: one cycle of Yin and Yang around every four or five seconds. Tai chi, therefore, seems to work at a level wholly in tune with our body's most basic rhythmic impulses, establishing harmony and calm throughout the entire nervous system.

But what about the conscious thought process itself? Tai chi relaxes the mind, of that there is no doubt no matter how unlikely this may seem to beginners struggling to learn the intricacies of the form. Ultimately, however, as you achieve a certain equanimity and detachment with the movements, the mind begins to function in a far more relaxed mode. This can, in fact, be measured by the frequency of electrical activity in the brain and is called the 'alpha state', in which the brain vibrates at a frequency of around 10 Hz. A similar frequency occurs just before we drop off to sleep or just as we are waking and is also achieved through the practice of meditation and yoga. The interesting thing is that during this and other highly relaxed states, there is a measurable increase in the formation of connective tissues between the brain cells, thereby enhancing our mental faculties at a very deep level.

The learning of the form not only improves our physical and mental co-ordination, it also provides us with what scientists call an 'enriched environment' – in other words, a stimulating activity to challenge our intelligence. Experiments have clearly demonstrated that an enriched environment and the repeated chemical boost we get within the brain itself from the process of problem solving also enhances the growth of connective tissue in the brain. Perhaps this is why those who regularly practise tai chi report increased mental clarity, along with better judgement and anticipation in their daily affairs.

# *Food and how to deal with it*

The constant emphasis in tai chi of turning from the centre and rotating the waist is enormously helpful for maintaining the health of the digestive system and bowels. This, together with the efficient descending of the diaphragm during inhalation, gently massages the intestines, liver and kidneys and promotes a healthy blood supply to all the abdominal organs.

Gastrointestinal disorders such as irritable bowel syndrome or peptic and duodenal ulcers benefit from the calming effect tai chi has on the digestive system and on the autonomic nervous system that controls its activity.

Cloudy Hands is renowned for its beneficial effects on the stomach. Diagonal Flying and Play Guitar are also considered helpful, while the Single Whip and Squatting Single Whip (Snake Creeps Down) benefit the liver in particular via the gentle bearing down pressure exerted upon it by the right rib cage. All toe stances and toe kicks stimulate the Spleen and Stomach acu-channels in the front of the leg and foot, aiding the digestive process and assisting with the correct assimilation of fluids into the body.

Of course, a good digestive system depends greatly on what you eat. Tai chi philosophy urges us to reflect on the Yin and Yang aspects of food so that we balance our intake with our environment and with the seasons. For instance, too many cold or raw foods (Yin) during the winter (Yin season) is bad news, as would be too many heat producing foods (Yang) during the summer. Skipping breakfast, particularly in winter when the stomach needs warming, is particularly unwise in terms of TCM, as are crash diets or lengthy fasts. And of course, heavily processed or junk foods need to be avoided, being poor in natural levels of chi and also often containing high levels of sugar, salt and artificial flavourings and colours, all of which use up considerable energy as the body struggles to eliminate them from the system.

> **66** *If the body is healthy, it can easily assimilate the stress of modern living and even find it a creative challenge.* **99**
> Mantak Chia

# Bones

A strong skeletal system is dependent on a good blood supply to the joints and on a healthy bone marrow which, in turn, helps manufacture the precious white blood cells that fight viruses and bacterial infection. Tai chi, in fact, is legendary in its ability to enhance the quality of the bone marrow via the TCM Kidney system. The chi is thought to somehow permeate the marrow, building up great resilience over a period of time. It was said of Cheng Man Ching that his arms felt like iron bars wrapped in cotton wool. This is a rare individual, of course, but it is an indication of what changes can be wrought in exceptional circumstances.

Those of us who work a lot with our hands and fingers will appreciate the relaxed rotation and flexing movements of the hands in tai chi, for stiffness can easily build up in the hands. This is apparent not only in well-known diseases like arthritis and rheumatism but also with modern illnesses such as carpal tunnel syndrome, brought about by continual keyboard operating.

# Muscles

Tai chi won't give you big muscles. But it will tone them up wonderfully. Good muscle tone depends on exercise and on an efficient blood supply and tai chi provides both of these. The ligaments and tendons that connect the muscles to the bones are strengthened with regular practice, particularly those of the legs and abdominal region, all of which increases our flexibility and ability to resist and cope with injury and strain. Moreover, those looking for a streamlining effect will find that because the *gluteus maximus* and other muscles of the behind are in constant use during the form, the backside gradually becomes firmer, as do also the thighs and calves, after several months of practice, while the constant turning of the body can also help to trim up the waistline.

The Opening sequence of the form, because of its symmetry and equal weight distribution, is said to benefit the internal muscular system by encouraging the proper placement and alignment of the body tissue. The Opening sequence can therefore be repeated several times, very slowly, for those interested in this possibility. It then becomes a kind of chi kung exercise (see Chapter 8).

# Glands

Most, if not all, of our bodily functions rely on chemical and hormonal stimuli and it is the endocrine glands of the body that are responsible for these. There are several major glands and we need them all. The thymus gland, located in the chest, plays a significant role in maintaining the immune system, while the adrenals, in the small of the back, produce chemicals that provide stamina, reduce inflammation and regulate blood pressure. The combination of tai chi movement and breathing, along with the constant emphasis on the chest, lower back and abdominal areas, is thought to stimulate both these glands. Meanwhile, the efficient flow of blood to the brain, promoted by relaxed shoulders and neck, naturally assists the pituitary and pineal glands which are responsible for growth and for regulation of the sexual and reproductive systems.

It is known that the glands of the body – especially the thymus – thrive in a happy individual, but they function poorly in those who are depressed. Probably, therefore, tai chi's greatest contribution in terms of maintaining a healthy immune system is in the calming and positive attitude developed by those who practise the form regularly.

# Urinary and reproductive systems

As we have seen, tai chi promotes the basic Kidney chi of the body, which in turn greatly facilitates the efficiency of all the reproductive organs, helping to maintain sexual vitality and fertility. The increased mobility and blood supply to the lower abdomen naturally also has a positive effect on the urinary system. Crescent Kick and all twisting and opening movements, such as Four Corners, are excellent for strengthening the internal muscles of the urinary and reproductive systems and for clearing congestion – recurring infections in the urinary system often being the result of congestion and stagnation of energy.

# Sex

Bearing in mind the Yellow Emperor and his hundred wives, the question must be asked: does tai chi make you sexier? Well, those who are fit and healthy are usually attractive to others, for obvious reasons – so yes, maybe tai chi does help. Moreover, tai chi and allied Taoist practices generate considerable vital energy which can be directed towards sexual capacity, if that's what you want – although by so doing, you can very quickly deplete your basic levels of chi. Most advanced practitioners of tai chi therefore are mindful of the Taoist teaching on sexual matters, which urges moderation. This is particularly important for men. Males loose much of their vital Kidney chi through ejaculation. Women fare much better in this respect, since the female orgasm is not considered to be debilitating. Women do, however, tend to lose their chi through menstruation and childbirth.

Regarding the controversial topic of male sexuality, therefore, teachers and writers in the fields of oriental philosophy and medicine have always urged the conservation of semen whenever reasonably possible, even during sexual activity. This is thought not only to conserve the chi but also, with the help of a partner, to help generate it internally. Once again, moderation and balance are the keywords here, as in so much of life.

It is hoped that this chapter has provided some insight into the intimate relationship between tai chi and our bodily processes. Tai chi is not like most other exercise systems where you are urged to run around endlessly, getting hot and irritable. Rather, it is about looking after your entire being, at all levels. And therefore, it is to the world of the mind and that most elusive entity, the spirit, that we will turn next.

> 66 *T'ai Chi Ch'uan brings the physical, emotional, mental, and spiritual energies into alignment once again as undivided oneness.* 99
>
> Michael Page

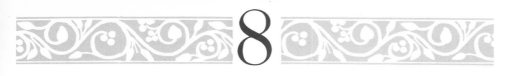

# 8

# BODY, MIND AND SPIRIT

## *Finding a teacher*

I hope this book has inspired you to go out and join a tai chi class or to find a teacher. Perhaps you are already attending evening classes or a formal school for tai chi, in which case it is pretty likely you are doing something similar to what is laid out in these pages. Yang style tai chi is very popular at the present time. But there are, of course, many variations of style and of emphasis even here. Some instructors, for example, teach tai chi wholly for its martial aspects and in so doing may fail to balance this with a transmission of the vital qualities of relaxation, calm and humility, all central to the Taoist tradition. Others might teach it entirely for its beauty and gracefulness and as a consequence may fail to generate real energy or any measure of strength in their pupils. These are the two extremes and, thankfully, you won't encounter them too often.

Look for balance, therefore, in this area as much as in any other. Also don't be anxious about asking your would-be teacher what precisely he or she intends to teach. You have every right to this information, especially if you are going to part with hard-earned cash. A good tai chi teacher will always be prepared to answer your questions and will not try to make you look small or hold you back from reaching the same level, in time, as they have reached themselves. A good teacher is also usually broad-minded and cheerful. The moment you encounter anybody who needs to justify their own standards by denigrating the work of others, you should proceed only with great caution. Those who have truly found the Tao in their lives realise the richness and depth of tai chi and will never put their own preferences and individual specialities over and above anybody else's.

And now for the transmission of a great secret. Often pupils search the world over for the magic 'touch of the master' or just the right word at the right time that will transform their lives. Often they wait for decades for the one vital crumb of information that will take them to the heights of enlightenment and skill in their chosen art – tai chi or anything else. Yet so often they are disappointed and the reason is very simple. They have overlooked the one really important principle that is at the very heart of excellence, a principle that can be described in just one simple word: Practice.

Just keep doing it – don't give up! Certainly you will need an instructor at various times, especially during the early days. Most students go through several until they find the right one. But unless you are priming yourself to become a super-human fighting machine, the basic techniques of tai chi – despite what many will tell you – are straightforward and easy to learn. Then it is mostly a matter of getting on with it and adhering to daily practice and study. That is the great secret – and it is all there, quite literally in your own hands.

> 66 *Overcoming others requires force*
> *Overcoming the self needs strength*
> *He who knows he has enough is rich* 99
>
> Tao Te Ching

# Between heaven and earth

By this stage, the two great polarities of Yang and Yin will feel more real for you, as you know where to find them in your tai chi movements and in your breathing also. But Yang and Yin do not stop there and the following table may help to broaden this concept a little, for the contemplation and realisation of these forces through the Tai Chi is ultimately a celebration of all nature and of our place within it (Fig. 10).

Helpful and interesting as such tables of correspondences are, you will probably have realised by now that everything in this respect is relative. A candle is Yang compared to a glow-worm, but Yin compared to the brilliance of the sun. And perhaps nowhere is this subtle relativity expressed with more skill and insight than in the Taoist arts. Here, the relative strengths and inter-relationships of the Yang and the Yin can be discerned constantly – in the empty spaces, for example, that so many drawings and paintings contain, contrasting with but somehow also supporting the more tangible contents of the picture. In Taoist poetry, also, renowned for its brevity, it is often what is *unsaid* that creates the meaning to the verses, rather than the words themselves.

In your tai chi work, too, this concept can be a rich source of inventiveness and spontaneity. Try doing a very Yin form sometime or a very quick and forceful Yang one. Or contemplate the Yang within a Yin form – only very slightly Yang. The breath can also be revisited in this respect. The inhalation can be Yin if you are doing the tai chi form in the usual way, but Yang if you are engaged in some forms of passive meditation or pure contemplation of the movement of internal energy.

> 66 *When the breath wanders, the mind is unsteady, but when the*
> *breath is still, so is the mind still.* 99
>
> Pradipika

| | |
|---|---|
| Positive | Negative |
| Light | Dark |
| Day | Night |
| Summer | Winter |
| Spring | Autumn |
| Dry | Moist |
| Warm | Cool |
| Expansion | Contraction |
| Forward | Reverse |
| Active | Meditative |
| Spirit | Matter |
| Firm | Yielding |
| Analytical | Intuitive |
| Fiery | Watery |
| Surface | Depth |
| Conscious | Unconscious |
| Extraverted | Introverted |
| Forthright | Reserved |
| From above | From below |
| Dispersal | Renewal |

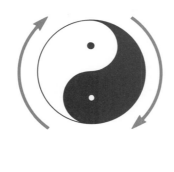

*Fig. 10   The qualities of Yang and Yin*

# Chi Kung

Closely allied to tai chi practice, and certainly predating it by many centuries, is the widespread practice of Chi Kung, the circulation and cultivation of chi through breathing and concentration. It is an amazingly complex area and if it is true that there are several, if not dozens, of different styles and variations within the world of tai chi, then in the closely related sphere of chi kung there are probably hundreds!

Chi Kung is usually, though not always, done standing and body movement is kept to a minimum. One of the most basic styles, especially suitable for those beginning tai chi, is shown here (Fig. 11). The feet are parallel, just a little more than shoulder width apart, the arms extended out in front of the chest as though embracing a large tree. The straight spine, the gently tucked in sacrum, the rounded aspect of the arms will all be familiar. You can think of it as tai chi without movement. Try it for a few minutes, perhaps at the beginning or at the end of your tai chi form. Keep the knees apart, 'spiralled out' like sitting on a horse. Sink down and think of your roots, the body itself suspended from above by that golden thread – upright between heaven and earth, between Yang and Yin, spirit and matter, the centre of its own universe.

Breathe deeply into the abdomen and be aware of the Tan Tien. Think of Yang energy and light as you breathe in and imagine a tiny golden ember smouldering away there. Every time you inhale, you fan it so it glows brighter. Then, as you breathe out, let the energy it produces spread throughtout your entire body. Keep the breath deep, long and even. Let it, and the movement of energy in the Tan Tien, fill your consciousness entirely.

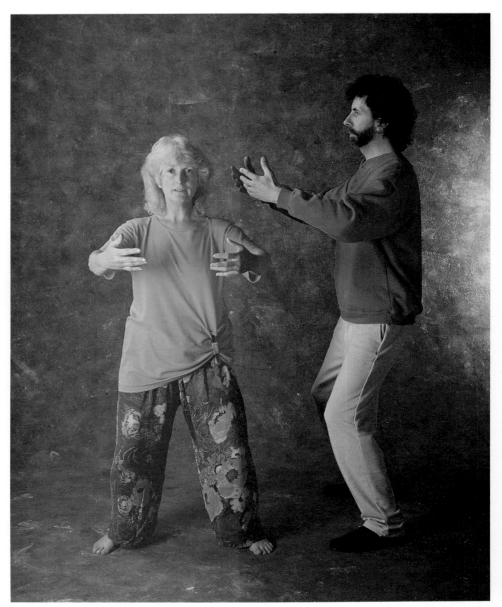

*Fig. 11   Chi Kung posture*

Later, try concentrating the feeling of energy into the spine, from where it rises to the shoulders, then down the arms. Let it connect down through the legs, to meet with the earth chi beneath your feet, or at a place on the sole of each foot called – very aptly – the 'Bubbling Spring'. Eventually, try letting it climb all the way up to the top of the head and then down the front again, via the forehead, throat, chest and abdomen, and returning to the Tan Tien – a circle of energy that transmits lifegiving chi to all the organs of the body in endless cycles of generation (Yang) and storage (Yin).

If at this stage, you place the tip of your tongue lightly against the roof of your mouth – as if saying the letter 'L' – it will greatly facilitate the flow of chi. This 'circuit' of energy is also a good safety precaution. Chi naturally likes to rise and if it gets lodged in the head it can cause problems including high blood pressure and headaches, and so this technique of circling the energy back down is particularly valuable.

The Chi Kung position should be held for a reasonable length of time, say at least two minutes at first, building up to as long as you wish later on. Up to 15 minutes is possible with practice. A variation on this position is to simply lower the arms down to the level of the solar plexus – a welcome change, after a while, as the arms start to tire.

# The five elements: pathways between body and mind

Any overview of tai chi philosophy would not be complete without a look at the five elements. The elements, as such, are not unique to China, of course. Every great culture has classified the natural forces of their environment into four or five universal categories. The Greeks, the American Indians, the brilliant artists and humanists of the European Renaissance, they all had their elemental forces. The Taoists recognise five elements: Fire, Earth, Metal, Water and Wood.

The term 'element' in the scientific sense usually means a particular atomic configuration these days and this can lead those of a purely orthodox persuasion to look down their noses somewhat at what they see as a primitive attempt to classify matter into its respective parts. But nothing could be further from the truth. The classical elements of antiquity go far beyond a mere preoccupation with matter. They are, in fact, a means of contemplating and understanding aspects of the whole environment – earth, sky, water, spirit, fire and energy, life and death, great and powerful forces to which the people of those times felt themselves both mentally and physically united, a kind of attachment to which those of us practising tai chi should also aspire, perhaps.

Consequently, and because of their pleasingly abstract quality, the elements have always been applicable to the field of medicine – and, indeed, still are – furnishing the practitioner of oriental medicine with an invaluable guide through the otherwise impenetrable complexity of the human body and the world around it. Fire, Earth, Metal, Water and Wood are all to be found in an energetic sense within the various organs and systems of the human body. Moreover, each element has a Yang and a Yin aspect, and there are Fire organs, such as the Heart, or Water organs, such as the Kidneys, as the following brief tour through the elements will show (Fig. 12).

| Wood | Fire | Earth | Metal | Water |
|------|------|-------|-------|-------|
| Spring | Summer | Late Summer | Autumn | Winter |
| Germination | Growth | Ripening | Harvest | Storage |
| East | South | Centre | West | North |
| Wind | Heat | Dampness | Dryness | Cold |
| Green | Red | Yellow | White | Black/Blue |
| Liver | Heart | Spleen | Lungs | Kidneys |
| Eyes | Tongue | Mouth | Nose | Ears |
| Anger | Elation | Pensiveness | Grief | Fear |
| Shouting | Laughing | Singing | Weeping | Groaning |
| Forest | Heath | Fields | Clouds | Rivers/Sea |
| Life | Sunshine | Soil | Minerals | Rainfall |
| Creativity | Inspiration | Common Sense | Melancholy | Contemplation |

*Fig. 12   Attributes of the five elements*

When the elements are working together, we are healthy; the body and mind act as a meaningful and dynamic whole. If, however, one element or organ becomes weak or overactive, the others will tend to compensate, which is all right for a while but if the imbalance continues, illness will arise.

For those of you trained in western physiology, it is helpful to understand that in oriental medicine the organs are described by their function throughout the whole body rather than by their mere physical structure or anatomical location. Each one, moreover, will borrow from and lend energy to neighbouring elements or organs, each affecting the other in endless cycles or creativity and dissolution. The cycles of interchange are described neatly by arranging the elements on a five-pointed star, enclosed by a circle. The giving or creative cycle is ranged around the circle, while the controlling or destructive cycle is shown by the internal star (Fig. 13).

It is easy to imagine how the Taoists first perceived these cycles in the natural world around them. Take time yourself to contemplate how they work out in any area of experience you care to apply them to. Think of the seasons; think of the cycles in nature and human affairs – it is a wonderful meditation in itself. Try also looking in depth at one element – say, one each week. Let it become a special part of your life for that

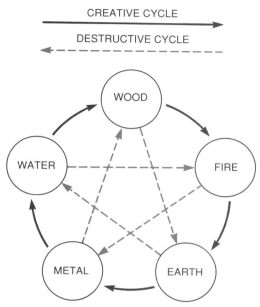

CREATIVE CYCLE

DESTRUCTIVE CYCLE

*Fig. 13   Creative and destructive cycles and the five element star*

period of time. Collect items from nature that exemplify that element – stones, shells, feathers and so on. Visit some water, the sea or a river; visit the woods; contemplate fire in all its manifestations; take up work in a garden.

Thus, through tai chi practice and its related studies we find not only a highly effective means of maintaining health through working on the physical body, but also are able to effect change on a far more powerful energetic level. It is a widely held view in oriental medicine that if the body is balanced so too will be the mind and, ultimately, the spirit. 'Spirit' is a strange word in our modern society. Many will refuse to recognise its existence and question the worth of pursuing such a vague and possibly illusory goal. The only reply to such cynicism is to continue with the tai chi – keep trying, keep working at it and eventually the answer will be found.

# *Taoism*

The Chinese philosophy of Taoism (pronounced 'Daoism', by the way) has always remained something which has to be experienced with the mind or heart, rather than the intellect. Of all belief systems or cultural practices throughout the world, Taoism is possibly unique in its refusal to be pinned down or classified. The main text on Taoism, the *Tao Te Ching*, written sometime around the sixth century BC when Taoism was already an old and venerable subject, has the clue to this elusive quality set forth in the very opening lines:

*The Tao that can be told is not the eternal Tao.*
*The name that can be named is not the eternal name.*
*The nameless is the beginning of heaven and earth.*

What the author, Lao Tsu, is referring to here is the source of existence. The Tao precedes the Tai Chi, therefore, in the great scheme of things, the order of creation which, like the five elements, is evident in everything around us (Fig. 14).

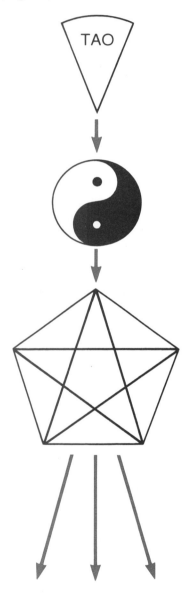

*Fig. 14   The creation tree*

The great Tao is clearly something beyond our experience and therefore beyond our powers of description. However, every living thing has its own smaller, more personal tao – written with a small 't' – its own path or purpose in life. The central idea of Taoism is that when we, as individuals, realise our own individual tao, it then becomes indivisible with the greater, universal Tao. Finding one's own 'way' means realising what is essential in one's life. It might be exhilarating to realise this or it could be painful.

Whatever the outcome, the Way is begun with the integration of Yang and Yin, the realisation of the Tai Chi in one's own life. After that, one simply waits for the tao to express itself. In this respect, the qualities that have been prized by the Taoists, such as spontaneity, non-violence, humility and detachment, can help us to overcome the ego and the endless desire for power and self-importance, so valued by our society yet which can never be really satisfied. Through these qualities a state of peace and harmony gradually arises, by which we can find the unifying principle of the Tao in the world about us as well as within our own hearts.

In this sense, it is not the destination but the journey which is of importance. You can view your tai chi practice, therefore, as symbolic of the journey to find the Tao. It then becomes synonymous with the archetypal 'Quest' or search so often described in great literature or fable. It is the Grail, the heroic journey, the battle for understanding. When viewed in this light, even the martial aspect of tai chi becomes a symbol for something far greater. Thus, in the Tao are all things reconciled.

You have now come to the end of this book. It is not intended to be an exhaustive summary of the subject. A thousand books could not even begin to do that. It is a signpost, that's all, and the journey lies ahead. I cannot tell you where it will lead for it is *your* journey, not mine or anybody else's. It is your tao and yours alone.

There is an old Chinese saying: 'If you cannot find it within yourself, where will you go for it?'. Have faith in your own powers, therefore. And may all good fortune be with you.

> 66 *Just as the path of the eagle in the air and the path of the snake are invisible, so also is the path of the sage.* 99
>
> Buddha

*Composite illustration of the sequence*

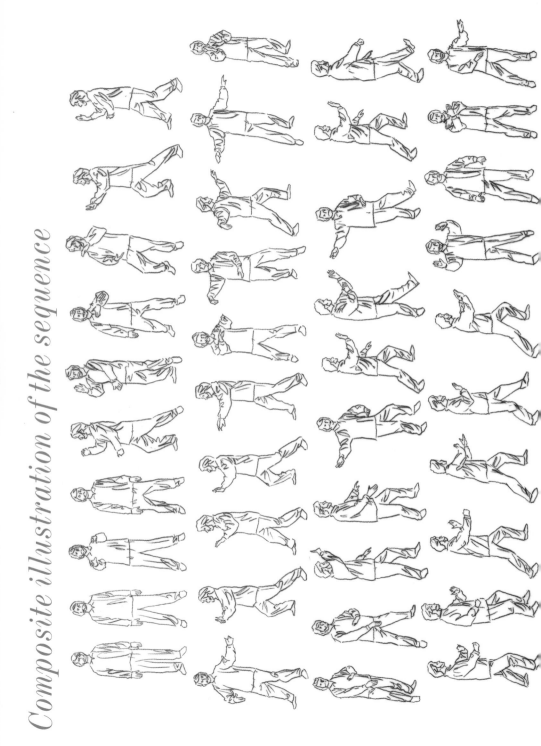

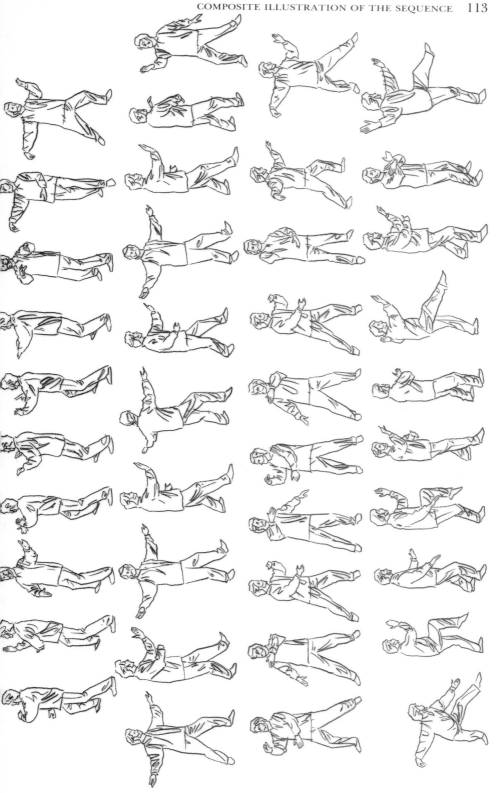

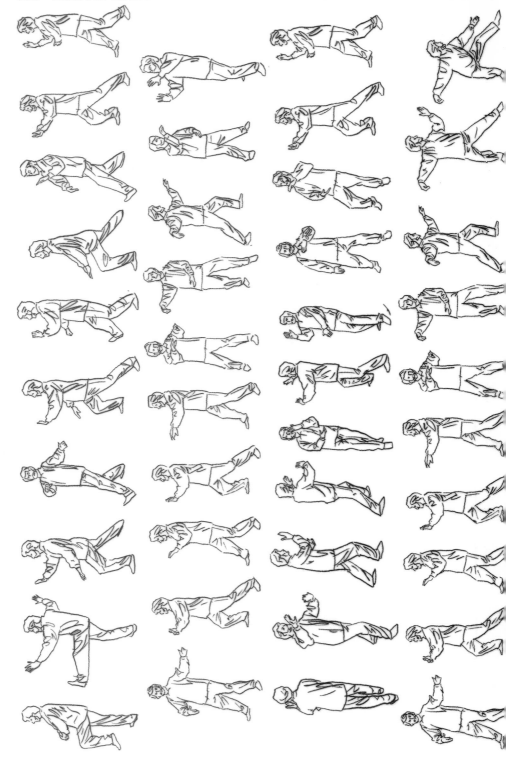

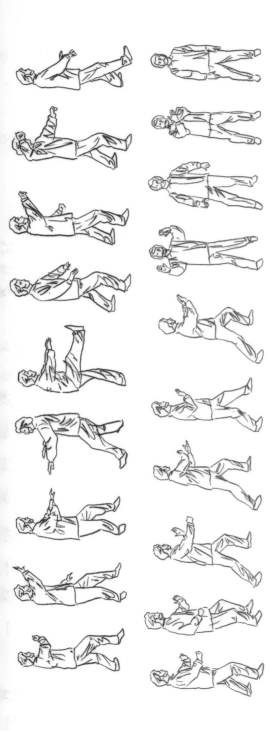

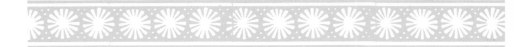

# FURTHER READING

Ch'ing Cheng Man, *Cheng Tzu's Thirteen Treatises on T'ai Chi Ch'uan*, North Atlantic Books, USA, 1985
Hass, E.M., *Staying Healthy with the Seasons*, Celestial Arts, California, 1981
Klein, Bob, *Movements of Magic*, Newcastle Publishing Co., USA
Page, Michael, *The Tao of Power*, Green Print, 1989
Tsu, Lao, *Tao Te Ching*, trs. Gia-Fu Feng and Jane English, Wildwood House, 1973
Wing, R.L., *The Illustrated I Ching*, Aquarian Press, London, 1987

# USEFUL ADDRESSES

There is no single umbrella organisation representing all of tai chi and the diversity of the subject probably means there never will be. But for anyone seeking good quality, expert instruction the following groups would certainly be of use:

British T'ai Chi Chuan Association and London T'ai Chi Academy
7 Upper Wimpole Street
London W1M 7TD
(Tel: 071–251 4076)

International Tai Chi Chuan Association
Studio 8
People's Hall
91/97 Freston Road
London W11

Prospective students should also inquire at their local Adult Education Centre (telephone number in the phone book, or prospectus from the local library) to see if it offers classes in tai chi. Many now do. These are ideal for beginners and are excellent value for money.